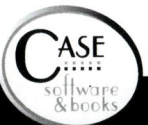

Laboratory Assessment of Nutritional Status:
Bridging Theory & Practice

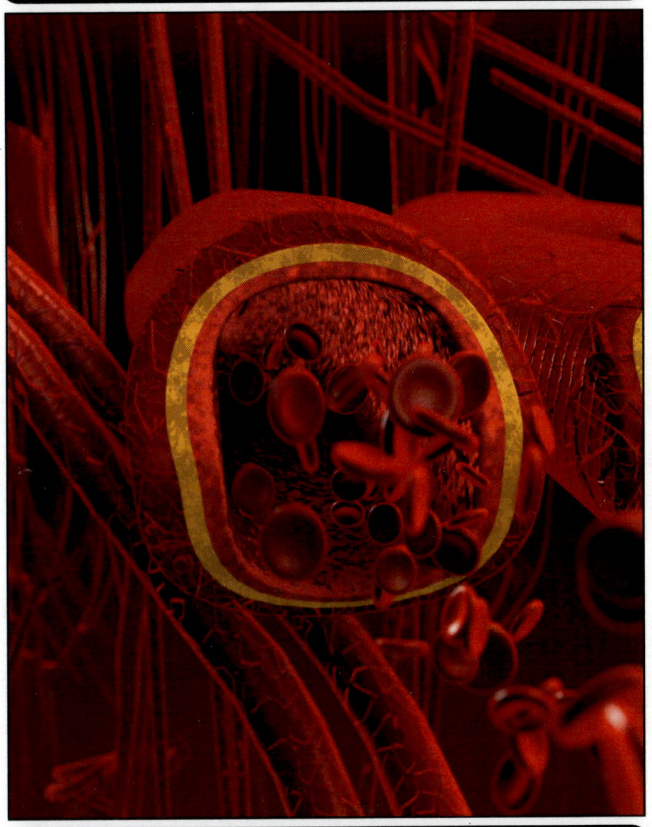

Mary D. Litchford, PhD, RDN, LDN

Copyright © 2011 with 6.11 updates, CASE Software
ISBN #978-1-880989-95-1

Library of Congress Control Number
2010902479

MARY D. LITCHFORD, PHD, RDN, LDN
Greensboro, NC 27410
mdlphd@casesoftware.com
www.CASEsoftware.com

All rights reserved. No part of this book may be reproduced by any graphic, mechanical, photographic or electronic process, or in the form of phonographic recording or otherwise copied for public or private use without written permission from the publisher.

NOTICE

Health care is an ever-changing field. Readers are advised to check the most current product information provided by the manufacturer to verify all reference values and medication-laboratory test interactions. Neither the publisher nor the author assume any liability for any injury and/or damage to persons or property arising from this publication.

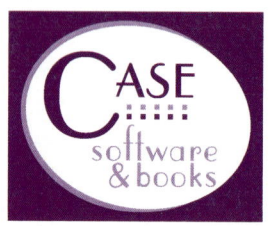

GREENSBORO, NC
www.CASEsoftware.com

LABORATORY ASSESSMENT OF NUTRITIONAL STATUS:
BRIDGING THEORY & PRACTICE

PREFACE

New technologies and innovative processes generate new information giving the practitioner a greater understanding of the cascade of events from diagnosis through treatment and outcomes. The Nutrition Care Process (NCP) is an innovative process in which nutrition care indicators are clustered together to identify nutrition diagnoses. Laboratory data remains one of the key components of the assessment section and is often incorporated into the PES statements.

Changes in laboratory values reflect changes in medical condition, but not always nutritional status. Be alert to all the factors that contribute to changes in laboratory values. Changes in nutritional status mean the plan of care is achieving the expected outcomes or it is not achieving the expected outcomes. Improving nutritional status usually means shorter hospital stays, fewer complications and speedier wound healing after surgery. Using laboratory assessment to document the positive impact of the medical nutrition therapy demonstrates the benefits of our professional expertise to the medical team.

Laboratory Assessment of Nutritional Status: Bridging Theory & Practice provides the user an essential reference for many clinically relevant laboratory tests used in nutritional assessment. One feature of this reference is its consistent and easy to use format. Each laboratory test is listed in alphabetical order to allow the user to locate tests quickly. An additional resource is the companion CE course with instructional case studies available online or on CD ROM approved by the

Commission on Dietetic Registration for 14 CE units at Level III. It is available from CASE Software & Books, casesoftware.com. Other professional reference books and CPE courses available from CASE Software & Books:

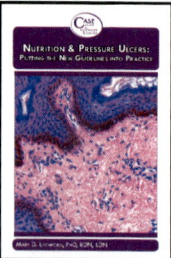

Nutrition & Pressure Ulcers: Putting the New Guidelines into Practice

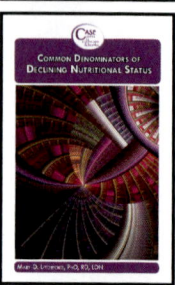

Common Denominators of Declining Nutritional Status

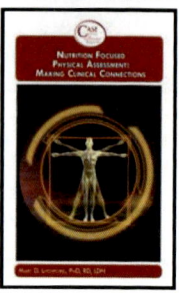

Nutrition Focused Physical Assessment: Making Clinical Connections

Many new research studies and technological advances are constantly reshaping the field of medicine. We welcome comments from users of this book so that we can provide useful relevant laboratory test information to users of future editions.

Mary D. Litchford, PhD, RDN, LDN

ABOUT THE AUTHOR

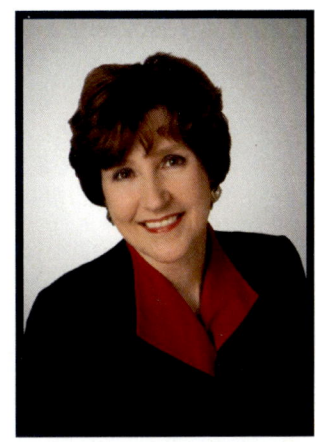

Mary D. Litchford PhD, RDN, LDN is an acclaimed author and speaker on a wide variety of nutrition and healthcare topics. She holds a masters degree in nutrition from the University of Tennessee-Knoxville and a doctorate of philosophy from the University of North Carolina-Greensboro. Dr. Litchford works as a medical-legal expert witness and consultant to the healthcare industry. She has received numerous life-time achievement awards for her professional contributions.

Dr. Litchford is president of CASE Software & Books. She has authored numerous advanced level CPE courses for nutrition professionals. For product information, contact CASE Software & Books, www.casesoftware.com.

Table of Contents

Introduction & Objectives	11
Overview	14
Implications of Selected Laboratory Tests	15
Changes in Nutritional Status	15
Impact of Inflammation	16
Reference Standards	18
Equipment	18
Considerations for Requesting Laboratory Tests	19
Communication of Results	20
Clinical Laboratory Values	20
Implications for Practice	26
Biochemical Assessment of Nutritional Status:	
Blood	27
Urine	28
Assessment of Hydration Status	29
Assessment of Protein Status	35
Nutritional Anemias	37
Review Questions for Critical Thinking	52
Laboratory Reference	
Alanine Aminotransferase	53
Alkaline Phosphatase	58
Ammonia, Blood	63
Apolipoprotein A&B	66
Apo a-1/Apo b Ratio	66
Lipoprotein (a)	66
Apolipoprotein E	66
Arterial Blood Gases	72
Aspartate Aminotransferase	79
Bilirubin, Blood & Urine	86
Blood Urea Nitrogen	93
C-Reactive Protein	98
High Sensitivity C-Reactive Protein	98
Calcium, Blood	101
Calcium, Urine	106
Chloride	111
Cholesterol	114
LDL, HDL, VLDL	114

CORTISOL, BLOOD & URINE	122
CREATINE KINASE	125
CREATININE CLEARANCE	129
CREATININE, SERUM	132
CREATININE, URINE	136
ERYTHROCYTE SEDIMENTATION RATE	138
FERRITIN	141
FIBRINOGEN	145
FOLATE, SERUM, RBC FOLATE	147
GLUCOSE, BLOOD	151
GLUCOSE, POST PRANDIAL	161
GLUCOSE TOLERANCE TEST	164
GLUCOSE, URINE	168
GLUCOSE-6-PHOSPHATE DEHYDROGENASE	171
GLYCOSYLATED HEMOGLOBIN (A1C)	173
HEMATOCRIT OR PACKED CELL VOLUME (PCV)	178
HEMOGLOBIN	180
HOMOCYSTEINE	183
IRON LEVELS	186
SERUM FE, TIBC, TRANSFERRIN, TRANSFERRIN SATURATION	186
LACTIC DEHYDROGENASE	191
MAGNESIUM, SERUM & URINE	195
METHYL MALONIC ACID, SERUM & URINE	199
NATRIURETIC PEPTIDES	201
OSMOLALITY, SERUM	204
OSMOLALITY, URINE	206
PHOSPHATE	208
POTASSIUM, SERUM	212
POTASSIUM, URINE	218
PROTEIN, BLOOD	220
RBP, PAB, ALBUMIN, GLOBULIN, TOTAL PROTEIN	220
PROTEIN, URINE	233
TOTAL PROTEIN, ALBUMIN, MICROALBUMIN	233
PROTHROMBIN TIME & INTERNATIONAL NORMALIZED RATIO	238
RED BLOOD CELL INDICES	240
MCV, MCH, MCHC, RDW	240
RETICULOCYTE COUNT & RETICULOCYTE INDEX	244
SCHILLING B_{12} ABSORPTION TEST	247
SODIUM, SERUM	250
SODIUM, URINE	256
SPECIFIC GRAVITY, URINE	258

THIAMIN (B1)	259
THYROID FUNCTION TESTS	262
TSH, TRH, TBG, T$_4$, FREE T$_4$, FTI, T$_3$, FREE T$_3$	262
TRIGLYCERIDES	277
TROPONINS	280
VITAMIN A, RETINOL	281
VITAMIN B$_6$	284
VITAMIN B$_{12}$	286
VITAMIN D 25(OH)D	289
VITAMIN E	291
WHITE BLOOD CELL (WBC) & COUNT DIFFERENTIAL COUNT	293
ZINC	300
REFERENCES	302
INDEX	312

List of Tables

TABLE 1. SELECTED ACUTE PHASE PROTEINS	17
TABLE 2. SELECTED SI UNITS & CONVERSION TABLE FOR VALUES IN CLINICAL CHEMISTRY	21
TABLE 3. ABBREVIATIONS & UNITS OF MEASUREMENT	25
TABLE 4. LABORATORY SCREENING FOR DEHYDRATION	33
TABLE 5. LABORATORY SCREENING FOR OVERHYDRATION	35
TABLE 6. ANEMIAS ACCORDING TO RBC INDICES	43
TABLE 7. GUIDE TO ANEMIAS	51
TABLE 8. ARTERIAL BLOOD GASES (ABG) WITH ACID-BASE DISTURBANCES	75
TABLE 9. COMPENSATORY RESPONSES IN ACID-BASE DISTURBANCES	75
TABLE 10. DEFINITIONS OF HYPERCALCIURIA	106
TABLE 11. EXPECTED URINE CALCIUM RANGES	106
TABLE 12. HDL LEVELS & RISK FOR CORONARY ARTERY DISEASE	117
TABLE 13. MEAN ESTIMATED GFR RATES	130
TABLE 14. FERRITIN VS. SERUM FE IN DIFFERENT CONDITIONS	143
TABLE 15. INTERPRETATION OF FPG FOR DM SCREENING	153
TABLE 16. DM DIAGNOSTIC CRITERIA FOR NON-PREGNANT ADULTS	154
TABLE 17. DIAGNOSTIC CRITERIA FOR DM USING PPG	161
TABLE 18. DIAGNOSTIC CRITERIA FOR GDM	162
TABLE 19. DIAGNOSTIC CRITERIA FOR GDM USING GTT	165
TABLE 20. DIAGNOSTIC CRITERIA FOR DM USING A1C	173

TABLE 21. APPROXIMATE CORRELATION BETWEEN
    A1C & MPG   175
TABLE 22. SYMPTOMS ASSOCIATED WITH HYPERMAGNESEMIA   197
TABLE 23. PROTEIN ELECTROPHORESIS PATTERNS IN
    SPECIFIC DISEASES   231
TABLE 24. PATTERN OF LAB TEST RESULTS FOR
    THYROID DYSFUNCTION   264

INTRODUCTION & OBJECTIVES

Each generation of nutrition professionals takes the profession to higher levels of expertise in the medical nutrition therapy. Laboratory assessment of nutritional status is one area that has seen dramatic changes in utilization of data to support NCP and demonstrate the 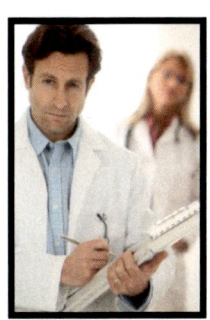 effectiveness of intervention strategies. Laboratory test results are tools for the nutrition professional to use while discussing the care needs of patients with other members of the medical team.

For purchasers of the self-study course, either online case studies or a CD-ROM of case studies, is included for application of concepts. Each case study provides a medical profile of the patient followed by a series of questions. Users receive specific, interactive assistance for any errors.

For the most effective use of the self-study course, users should have a clear understanding of interpreting abnormal patterns of laboratory values, medical physiology, common physiological changes that occur with injury, surgery or aging, disease processes and the relationship between changes in laboratory values and changes in general health.

LEARNING OBJECTIVES:

At the completion of this course, the successful learner will be able to:

- Discuss the role of inflammatory biomarkers as it relates to declining nutritional status.

- Assess laboratory test results for hydration status, protein status, nutritional anemia and other nutrition related disorders.
- Describe the relationship between laboratory test results and changes in nutritional status.
- Differentiate the role of medications and disease as each affects laboratory test results.
- Apply principles of Nutrition Care Process in the laboratory assessment of nutritional status

CDR Learning Codes that can apply to this course include 2100, 3000, 3020, 3060, 5000, 5010, 5020, 5030, 5040, 5050, 5080, 5090, 5100, 5230 or other applicable codes.

Information for Self-Study Course Participants
Online Users

Your confirmation email includes the computer links to the online case studies and competency testing. These links expire in TEN DAYS! Be sure to bookmark these links for later use. If you are unable to access the URL links when it is time to complete the case studies or competency testing, please contact us by email. We will resend the links.

Once you have read the text, apply your knowledge with the online case studies. Users are asked to respond to a variety of questions. The case studies provide feedback to the correctness of your answer. At the completion of each case study are your score and a list of study recommendations. Complete each case study and then take the online exam. You must score 70 percent on the competency exam to receive a Certificate of Completion. You may take the online exam more than once to achieve this benchmark. Once online users have passed the competency exam, please complete the Professional Continuing Education Survey and print your Certificate of Completion.

Hard Copy Users

Your order included a CD-ROM of case studies and a paper competency exam with answer sheet. Once you have read the text, apply your knowledge with the CD-ROM of case studies. Users are asked to respond to a variety of questions. The case studies provide feedback to the correctness of your answer. At the completion of each case study are your score and a list of study recommendations. Complete each case study and then take the paper competency exam. You must score 70 percent on the competency exam to receive a Certificate of Completion. Please complete the Professional Continuing Education Survey and either mail or fax your answer sheet and survey to the address on the answer sheet. Keep a copy of your answer sheet and Professional Continuing Education Survey for your records. A Certificate of Completion will be mailed to you within 10 working days. Please call or email us if you do not receive your Certificate of Completion within two weeks after it was mailed to CASE Software & Books. If you have a tight deadline to meet, we will be happy to fax your Certificate of Completion to you per your instructions.

Other Users:

If you purchased this course from a source other than CASE Software & Books, follow the instructions for completing the self-study course provided at the time of your purchase.

OVERVIEW

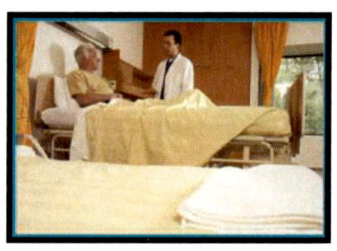

Nutrition Care Process (NCP) is a systemic problem-solving method for RDNs to use to think critically and make decisions to address nutrition problems. The goal is provide high quality care documented using standardized language.

All steps of NCP can incorporate laboratory values. In the Nutrition Assessment step, practitioners are to review data, cluster nutrition care indicators and identify standards by which the data will be compared. Next, determine the Nutrition Diagnosis. Under the clinical domain, biochemical section, are the nutrition diagnosis specifically related to changes in laboratory values. Laboratory values may be incorporated into PES statements in the signs and symptoms section as well. In the final step of NCP, Nutrition Monitoring and Evaluation, laboratory data may be useful to determine if Nutrition Diagnoses are resolved or new ones are present. It is important to remember that requesting more laboratory testing does not always equate with best practices. Centers for Medicare (CMS) F-tag 314, Comprehensive Assessment under nutrition, malnutrition & hydration deficits states:

> 'Although some laboratory tests may help clinicians evaluate nutritional issues in a resident with pressure ulcers, no laboratory test is specific or sensitive enough to warrant serial/repeated testing.
> Serum albumin, prealbumin and cholesterol may be useful to help establish overall prognosis; however, they may not correlate well with clinical observation of nutritional status.'

Incorporating laboratory assessment as a tool to assess nutrition status is supported in the research literature and used by other medical team members. ***Laboratory Assessment of Nutritional Status: Bridging Theory & Practice*** is a reference to assist the healthcare practitioner in documenting the role of medical nutrition therapy through NCP.

IMPLICATIONS OF SELECTED LABORATORY TESTS

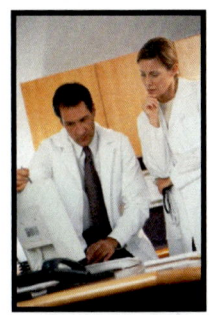

Test selections are based on subjective clinical judgement, national recommendations and evidenced-based medicine. Patient's knowledge of diagnostic screening tests may be from friends, family and the Internet. It is critical that patients understand that not all information on the Internet is reliable or pertinent to their unique medical status.

Not all tests are appropriate for all patients, i.e. creatinine excretion cannot be used to evaluate muscle mass in patients with renal failure because the test assumes normal renal function. Remember that the overall medical condition of the patient, the current medications, and the psychoneuroimmunology must be considered in the interpretation of laboratory tests.

CHANGES IN NUTRITIONAL STATUS

A single laboratory test may or may not reflect improved nutritional status once a medical nutrition therapy intervention program has begun. Changes in hydration status significantly affect the laboratory results. More than one laboratory test is required to accurately document changes in nutritional status. Using support data such as physical findings, changes in anthropometric data, reported symptoms and diet will increase confidence in laboratory results.

IMPACT OF INFLAMMATION

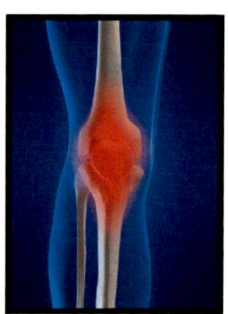

Interpreting laboratory tests must include the impact of inflammatory stress. There are two types of inflammation, acute or innate and chronic. Acute inflammation is a short-term process in which inflammatory mediators have short half lives and are quickly degraded. This occurs following injury, surgery or trauma. Chronic, inappropriate inflammation occurs when the immune response to injury is not extinguished. The persistent immune response acts like a slow burning fire that stimulates the synthesis of proinflammatory cytokines which promote erosion of lean body mass. Chronic inflammation is one of the hallmarks and underlying contributor to many diseases.

Inflammatory response occurs with or without infection. The classic signs are redness, swelling, pain, heat and loss of function. When the inflammation occurs in internal organs or structures, all the classic signs of inflammation may not be present. Inflammation triggers an immune response which initiates the release of both proinflammatory and anti-inflammatory cytokines. To combat the proinflammatory cytokines, the body must mobilize nutrient stores to produce acute phase proteins and T and B lymphocytes.

ACUTE PHASE PROTEINS

Acute phase proteins are either positive or negative. In the presence of inflammation, with or without infection, the synthesis of positive acute phase proteins increases dramatically at the expense of the negative acute phase proteins. The concentration of positive acute phase proteins increases by at least 25 percent following an inflammatory response. Values can increase to 1000 times normal. Some of the inflammatory markers are specific while others are non-specific to the source of inflammation. Tracking the positive acute phase proteins to determine when inflammatory process wanes may be misleading if inflammation improves in one area while other underlying areas of inflammation may be present. Table 1 categorizes selected acute phase proteins as either positive or negative.

Negative acute phase proteins plummet in the presence of inflammation. Levels decrease by at least 25 percent. For example, a 25 percent drop in an albumin of 3.0 g/dL would be 2.25 g/dL. The albumin does not evaporate or disintegrate. It simply shifts from the extravascular space to the plasma.

Table 1. Selected Acute Phase Proteins

Positive Acute Phase Proteins	Negative Acute Phase Proteins
■ C-reactive protein (CRP) ■ hs-CRP ■ Fibrinogen ■ Plasminogen-activator-inhibitor 1 (PAI-1) ■ Serum amyloid A ■ Ferritin ■ Ceruloplasmin	■ Albumin ■ Prealbumin ■ Transferrin ■ Insulin-like growth factor 1

Reference Standards

Standard laboratory reports are referenced using suggested normal or age-appropriate values. Remember that many reference standards were developed based upon clinical research using primarily young and middle aged adults. Clinical research on the very young and very old is limited. Reference standards may not apply to these age groups. This is of particular concern in assessing the growing elderly population because their norms appear to be slightly lower or higher than the standards, but the acceptable difference has yet to be defined. Some manufacturers of laboratory assay equipment have developed age reference standards using their databases. The director of your institution's laboratory will be able to assist you in evaluating the available database and in incorporating the equipment specific reference standards into the laboratory reports generated for each individual.

Equipment

The most accurate measure of changes in nutritional status is using laboratory results from the same institution. Comparing laboratory results from different institutions can be like comparing apples to oranges. Each institution establishes reference standards and laboratory procedures for each test as suggested by the manufacturer. Other sources of variation include equipment used, the degree of equipment calibration and the skill of the technician.

CONSIDERATIONS FOR REQUESTING LABORATORY TESTS

Historically, the physician made all healthcare diagnostic decisions exclusively. In managed care, the multidisciplinary teams work together to make diagnostic recommendations to improve outcomes. As a member of the health care team, it is important to know the clinical value of a test related to its sensitivity, its specificity, its predictive value and the incidence of the disease in the population tested.

Sensitivity refers to the ability of a test to correctly identify individual who truly have a disease. Specificity refers to the ability of a test to correctly identify those individuals who do not have the disease. Sensitivity and specificity do not change with different populations of ill and healthy patients. Predictive value refers to the ability of a screening test result to correctly identify the disease state. The predicative value of the same test can vary considerably with age, gender and geographic location.

As part of the critical thinking matrix of the NCP, it is vital that the nutrition professional consider the following questions when requesting additional laboratory tests.

1) Will the outcome actually change the nutrition plan of care?

If not, then why are you requesting the test be done?

2) Is the test cost-effective?

The cost of lab tests is based on a variety of factors including the volume of individual tests or panels of tests processed at the lab. Lab tests that must be sent to another lab to be processed are considerably more expensive than anything done in house.

3) Is your goal for the patient consistent with their treatment goals and advanced directives?

Be sure to talk with the patient or family to clarify purpose of more testing and how the results might change the plan of care Confirm that additional testing is desired.

COMMUNICATION OF RESULTS

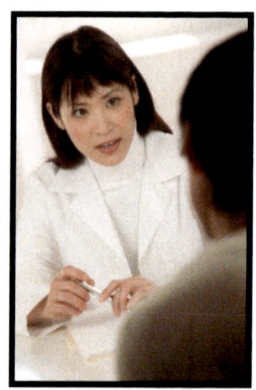

Numerous members of the health care team will be sharing the test results with the patient or family. Effective communication is at the heart of patient-center care and is crucial to achieve desired outcomes, prevent misunderstanding and help patients feel connected to the diagnostic process. Remember that the news may create emotional turmoil, shock and denial. Anxiety may persist for several days until the person has had time to assimilate the information. One of the ultimate goals of the NCP is to help the patient integrate the changes in health status into new life patterns.

CLINICAL LABORATORY VALUES

There are two systems for reporting clinical data either in conventional units or International Units (SI). The preferred method for reporting clinical laboratory data is in terms of International Units (SI Units). "SI Units" term is an abbreviation for le Système International d'Unités or International System. The reason for the change to SI units is to have an international standard for reporting research and medical data.

Laboratory Assessment of Nutritional Status: Bridging Theory & Practice provides both conventional units and SI units since both are used widely. Table 2 includes conversion factors for selected laboratory tests.

> **Conventional Units can be converted to SI Units using this formula:**
> Conventional Units x conversion factor = SI Unit
> **SI Units can be converted to Conventional Units using this formula:**
> SI Unit ÷ conversion factor = Conventional Unit

Table 2 provides conversion factors for selected values in Clinical Chemistry.

TABLE 2. SELECTED SI UNITS & CONVERSION TABLE FOR VALUES IN CLINICAL CHEMISTRY

Component	Conventional Reference values/ Units	Conversion factor	SI Reference Values/ Units
Alanine Aminotransferase (ALT) (S)	5-40 U/L	1.0	5-40 U/L
Albumin (S)	3.5-5.0 g/dL	10.0	35-50 g/L
Alkaline Phosphatase (S)	35-112 U/L	0.01667	0.5-2.0 μkat/L
Ammonia (vP)	10-80 mcg/dL	0.5909	6-47 μmol/L
Aspartate Aminotransferase (AST) (S)	0-35 U/L	0.01667	0.0-0.58 μkat/L
Bilirubin, total (S)	0.1-1.2 mg/dL	17.10	2-20 μmol/L

S = Serum, B = Blood, P = Plasma, U = Urine

TABLE 2. SELECTED SI UNITS & CONVERSION TABLE FOR VALUES IN CLINICAL CHEMISTRY

Component	Conventional Reference values/ Units	Conversion factor	SI Reference Values/ Units
Bilirubin, direct (S)	0.0-0.2 mg/dL	17.10	0.0-4.0 µmol/L
Calcium (S)	8.6-10.3 mg/dL	0.2495	2.15-2.57 mmol/L
Chloride (S)	98-108 mEq/L	1.00	98-108 mmol/L
Cholesterol (P)	<200 mg/dL	0.02586	<5.15 mmol/L
Creatinine (S) Males Females	0.6-1.2 mg/dL 0.5-1.1 mg/dL	88.40 88.40	53-106 µmol/L 44-97 µmol/L
Creatinine (U)	Variable g/24 hr	8.840	Variable mmol/L
Cyanocobalamin (S) (Vitamin B12)	250-950 pg/mL	0.7378	118-701 pmol/L
Ferritin (S) Males Females	29-438 ng/mL 9-219 ng/mL	1.00 1.00	29-438 µg/dL 9-219 µg/dL
Folate (S)	2.5-20 ng/mL	2.266	6-46 nmol/L
Glucose (P) fasting	70-100 mg/dL	0.05551	3.9-5.5 mmol/L
Hematocrit volume fraction female male	37-47% 42-52%	0.01 0.01	0.37-0.47 0.42-0.52
Hemoglobin (B) Male Female	14-18 g/dL 12-16 g/dL	0.6214 0.6214	8.7-11.2 mmol/L 7.4-9.9 mmol/L
Iron (S) Male Female	80-180 mcg/dL 60-160 mcg/dL	0.1791 0.1791	14-32 µmol/L 11-29 µmol/L

TABLE 2. SELECTED SI UNITS & CONVERSION TABLE FOR VALUES IN CLINICAL CHEMISTRY

Component	Conventional Reference values/Units	Conversion factor	SI Reference Values/Units
Iron binding capacity	230-410 mcg/dL	0.1791	41-73 µmol/L
Lactate dehydrogenase (S)	120-300 U/L	1	120-300 U/L
Lipoproteins (P) low density (LDL)	<100 mg/dL	0.02586	< 2.59 mmol/L
high density (HDL)	> 40 <60 mg/dL	0.02586	>1.0 < 1.55 mmol/L
Mean corpuscular hemoglobin concentration (MCH) mass	27-31 pg	1	27-31 pg
MCV (MCV)	80-100 um³ (microns³)	1	80-100 fL
Mean corpuscular hemoglobin concentration (MCHC)	32-36 %	0.01	0.32-0.36
Osmolality (P)	278-300 mOsm/kg H$_2$O	1.00	278-300 mmol/kg H$_2$O
Osmolality (U) Random	Varies mOsm/kg	1.00	Varies mmol/kg
Phosphate (S)	2.3-4.1 mg/dL	0.3229	0.75-1.35 mmol/L
Potassium ion (S)	3.7-5.1 mEq/L	1.00	3.7-5.1 mmol/L
Sodium ion (S)	134-142 mEq/L	1.00	134-142 mmol/L

TABLE 2. SELECTED SI UNITS & CONVERSION TABLE FOR VALUES IN CLINICAL CHEMISTRY

Component	Conventional Reference values/ Units	Conversion factor	SI Reference Values/ Units
Thyroid-stimulating hormone (TSH)	0-5 µIU/mL	1.0	0-5 mIU/L
Thyroxine T4 Male Female	4.0-12.0 mcg/dL 5.0-12.0 mcg/dL	12.87 12.87	51-154 nmol/L 64-154 nmol/L
Triiodothyronine T3	70-235 ng/mL	0.01536	1.1-3.6 nmol/L
Transferrin (S) Male Female	215-365 mg/dL 250-380 mg/dL	0.01 0.01	2.15-3.65 g/L 2.50-3.80 g/L
Triglycerides (S)	<100 mg/dL	0.01129	<1.13 mmol/L
Urea nitrogen (S)	6-25 mg/dL	0.3570	2.1-8.9 mmol/L

S = Serum, B = Blood, P = Plasma, U = Urine

Adapted from Fischbach, F A *Manual of Laboratory and Diagnostic Tests*, 8th ed. Philadelphia, PA, Lippincott, Williams & Wilkins

Laboratory Assessment of Nutritional Status: Bridging Theory & Practice uses a variety of standard abbreviations and units of measurement listed in Table 3. Many organizations are moving away from the use of lower case Greek letters such as µ for micro to avoid miscommunication. Please note that your institutional policy on standard abbreviations and units of measurement may vary.

TABLE 3. ABBREVIATIONS & UNITS OF MEASUREMENT

Abbreviation	Definition	Abbreviation	Definition
<	Less than	kg H$_2$O	Kilogram of water
≤	Less than or equal to	L	Liter
>	Greater than	m	Meter
≥	Greater than or equal to	m^2	Square meter
AU	Arbitrary units	m^3	Cubic meter
C	Celsius	mcg	Microgram
cc	Cubic centimeter	μmol	Micromole
cg	Centigram	mEq	Milliequivalent
cm	Centimeter	mEq/L	Milliequivalent per liter
cm H$_2$O	Centimeter of water	mg	Milligram
cu	Cubic	min	Minute
dL	Deciliter (100 mL)	mL	Milliliter
fl	Femtoliter	mm	Millimeter
fmol	Femtomole	mm^3	Cubic millimeter
g or gm	Gram	mM	Millimole
h	Hour	mm Hg	Millimeter of mercury
IU	International Unit	mm H$_2$O	Millimeter of water
ImU	International milliunit	mol	Mole
ImcU	International microunit	mmol	Millimole
IU	International Unit	mOsm	Milliosmole
K	Kilo	mμ	Millimicron
kat	Katal	mU	Milliunit
kg	Kilogram	mμ	Millimicron

25

LABORATORY ASSESSMENT OF NUTRITIONAL STATUS:
BRIDGING THEORY & PRACTICE

TABLE 3. ABBREVIATIONS & UNITS OF MEASUREMENT

Abbreviation	Definition	Abbreviation	Definition
μ^3	Cubic micron	ng	Nanogram
µKat	Microkatal	nm	Nanometer
µg	Microgram	nmol	Nanomole
µL	Microliter	Pa	Pascal
µm	Micrometer	pg	Picogram
μm^3	Cubic Micrometer	pL	Picoliter
µIU	Microinternational unit	pmol	Picomole
µmol	Micromole	sec	Second
µU	Microunit	SI Units	International System of Units
mV	Millivolt	U	Unit

IMPLICATIONS FOR PRACTICE

***Laboratory Assessment of Nutritional Status*: Bridging Theory & Practice** was designed to be used by RDNs, RNs, case managers, DTRs, CDMs and healthcare science students as a reference tool. It includes over 90 laboratory tests with a nutritional significance. Laboratory tests include normal values, critical values, nutritional significance, disease states that increase or decrease results and medications which may increase or decrease results. All laboratory values are listed in alphabetical order for easy reference. An index is provided for cross reference.

BIOCHEMICAL ASSESSMENT OF NUTRITIONAL STATUS

Biochemical assessment is an essential tool to assess the body's ability to convert food into body components. It is the foundation of the nutrition intervention program, one of the measuring sticks by which to evaluate its success and to predict medical outcomes.

National trends indicate a declining number of laboratory tests are being ordered in all areas of health care. This trend is a reflection of a better understanding of the predictive value of certain tests and cost-reduction programs nationwide. Assessment of physical and nutritional status is done primarily through physical assessment and observed dietary intake. Justification for ordering laboratory tests is based on observed clinical signs and symptoms.

Laboratory tests are based on analysis of blood and urine samples, which contain nutrients, enzymes and metabolites that reflect protein, vitamin and mineral status, presence of other components in body fluids. Common studies include enzymes, serum lipids, electrolyte levels, red and white blood cell counts, clotting factors and breakdown products such as urea nitrogen.

BLOOD

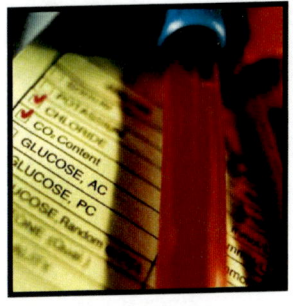

The total volume of blood in the human body is approximately 5-6 liters or 8 percent of body weight. Plasma is the fluid remaining after the cellular elements have been removed from the blood. Serum is obtained by clotting the blood before the removal of cells. The serum then does not contain the protein fibrinogen required for blood clotting.

The pH of the blood is in a range between 7.36 and 7.44. The buffer system helps to maintain the pH within this narrow range.

An increase or decrease in the cellular elements or constituents of the blood can be indicative of a nutritional deficiency, disease and acute or chronic blood loss. Blood analysis results are used for diagnosis as well as following the course of the deficiency, disease or recovery from injury or trauma.

Patients receiving blood transfusions have laboratory test results that reflect the nutritional status of the blood donor. The purpose of the transfusion is to replete the patient's body with key components. Interpretation of lab tests following a transfusion does not reflect the patient's true ability to convert food into body components.

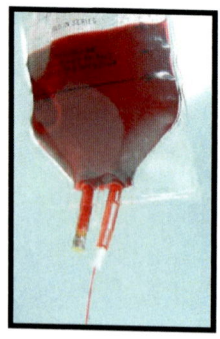

URINE

Urine is a mixture of water, inorganic salts and organic compounds. The major inorganic ions excreted are cations, sodium, potassium, calcium, magnesium and ammonium. The anions are chloride, phosphate and sulfate. The nitrogenous and non-nitrogenous organic compounds excreted in the urine are the waste products of metabolism. Water-soluble vitamins and their metabolites may be excreted in the urine. The volume of urine excreted is approximately 600 to 2500 mL per day. The normal pH range of urine is between 4.6 and 8.0 with an average of 6.0

(Pagana, 2009), depending on time of sampling and what food was consumed. The specific gravity of urine falls between 1.005 and 1.029 (Pagana, 2009), but can be affected by dehydration, renal disease, diabetes, fever and aging.

Urinalysis reports include remarks about the color, appearance and odor of the urine. Tests performed include pH, presence of protein, glucose, ketones, blood, and leukocyte esterase. The urine is examined microscopically for red and white blood cells (WBC), casts, crystals and bacteria. While nutritional assessment has focused primarily on blood analysis, some urine tests are included.

ASSESSMENT OF HYDRATION STATUS

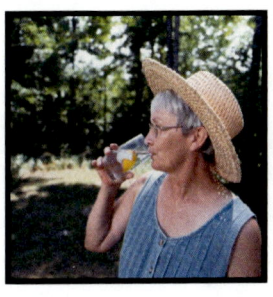

Disorders of fluid balance include dehydration and overhydration. Both present challenging physiological conditions that can be addressed using NCP. Inappropriate interventions can create additional problems.

Dehydration is the most common fluid electrolyte disorder of frail older adults living in community or institutional settings (Lavizzo-Mourey, 1988). Since no single measure has proved to be the 'gold standard' in the diagnosis of dehydration, it is often overlooked or misdiagnosed (Faes, 2007). Dehydration is a special concern for the hospitalized patient and long-term care resident. It is one of the most frequent diagnoses for admission to the hospital for patients 65 years and older. Mortality of patients with dehydration is high if not treated adequately and in some studies exceeds 50 percent (Bourdel-Marchesson, 2004). In terms of morbidity, several studies have shown an association between severe dehydration and poor mental function (Seymour, 1980; Wilson, 2003). Other studies found that dehydration was a significant risk factor for developing thromboembolic complications, infectious disease, kidney stones and obstipation (fecal impaction) (Embon, 1990; Wrenn, 1989).

Total body water accounts for about 60 percent of total body weight of middle-aged adults and about 45 – 50 percent of total body weight of elderly adults (Narins, 1994). The clinical significance of these numbers is that the elderly reach clinical dehydration faster than younger adults. Total body fluids decline in the elderly primarily because of a change in body composition. With age, older adults tend to lose lean muscle mass and gain fat. Lean muscle mass contains a higher percentage of water than fat which contains very little water. Changes in fluid balance in seniors can have a dramatic impact on their health and well-being (Chidester, 1997; Inouye, 1999; Rauscher, 2001; Welch, 1998).

Persons who are seriously ill and older adults tend to have a decreased thirst sensation due to confusion, an altered state of consciousness, or severe depression. Dehydration can occur during episodes of illness, fever, diaphoresis and inadequate replacement fluids. Fluid needs increase by 7 percent per degree of fever measured in Fahrenheit and by 12 percent per degree of fever measured in Celsius.

Early signs of dehydration include:
- Headaches
- Fatigue
- Loss of appetite
- Flushed skin
- Poor skin turgor
- Heat intolerance
- Lightheadedness
- Dry mouth and eyes
- Dark urine with strong odor(Kleiner, 1999)

Maintenance of fluid balance is essential to good health and recovery from surgery, illness or injury. Increased fluid losses are associated with:

- Chronic or acute infections
    - Fever
- GI losses
    - Vomiting
    - Diarrhea
    - Laxative abuse
    - Gastric drainage
    - Ileostomy
- Excessive urinary losses
    - Diuretics
    - Glycosuria
    - Diabetes insipidus
    - High-protein diet
- Environment
    - Elevated ambient temperature
    - Low humidity

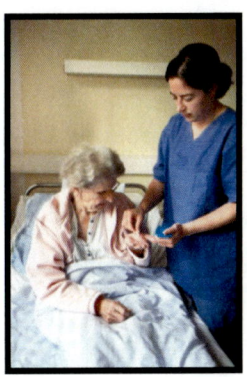

The decrease in body fluids causes reductions in both the extracellular and intracellular fluid compartments. Clinical manifestations of dehydration are closely related to intravascular volume depletion. Without treatment, dehydration progresses to hypovolemic shock, organ failure and death (Ellsbury, 2003).

Assessment for Dehydration

Assessment for dehydration in the hospitalized patient or long-term care resident involves:

- Physical assessment
- Recent history of food and fluid intake
- Laboratory assessment

During a dehydrated state, there is less water in the body. The concentration of blood constituents increases. The laboratory tests may present a misleading picture of the individual's nutritional status. There are three types of dehydration based on serum sodium:

- Hypertonic dehydration
- Isotonic dehydration
- Hypotonic dehydration

Hypertonic dehydration occurs when body water losses are greater than sodium losses. This can be due to reduced oral intake, excessive losses from sweating or prolonged high fever. The sodium concentration rises in the extracellular compartment, which draws water osmotically from the intracellular fluids. A summary of laboratory tests used to diagnose different types of dehydration follows on Table 4. Additional information about each laboratory test is in the next section of this text.

Isotonic dehydration occurs when the body loses equal amounts of sodium and water. Gastrointestinal disturbances causing extreme diarrhea and/or vomiting can trigger isotonic dehydration. This type of dehydration is often seen with food borne illness or severe bleeding. The serum sodium levels, serum osmolality and specific gravity levels are within normal ranges. These individuals are not thirsty and do not sense the need for more fluid. Both fluid and sodium are needed to rehydrate the patient. Refer to Table 4.

Hypotonic dehydration occurs when the body sodium loss exceeds water loss. This is sodium depletion or hyponatremia. It occurs in the patient who is taking diuretics, on sodium restricted diets, experiencing diarrhea or vomiting, has excessive sweating, a renal sodium-wasting syndrome or a combination of these contributors. There is typically a reduction in extracellular fluid volume. The laboratory tests indicate abnormally low serum sodium levels. Treatment includes giving water-electrolyte solutions to rehydrate the patient. Refer to Table 4.

TABLE 4. SCREENING FOR DEHYDRATION

Lab Test	Hypertonic	Isotonic	Hypotonic
Osmolality (S)	>Normal	WNL	< Normal
Sodium, (S)	> Normal	WNL	< Normal
Hemoglobin	> Normal	> Normal	> Normal
Hematocrit	> Normal	> Normal	> Normal
Albumin, (S)	> Normal	> Normal	> Normal
BUN	> Normal	> Normal	> Normal
Urine Specific Gravity	> Normal	> Normal	< Normal

Key: WNL= within normal limits

Assessment for Overhydration

Overhydration occurs when there is an increase in the extracellular fluid volume. The fluid shifts from the extracellular compartment to the interstitial fluid compartment. This is called edema and is typically caused by one of these mechanisms:

- ↑ capillary hydrostatic pressure (CHF)
- ↓ colloid osmotic pressure (hypoalbuminemia)
- ↑ capillary permeability (inflammation)
- Lymphatic obstruction (following surgery)
- Organ failure (kidney or liver)
- ↓ physical activity

Overhydration is categorized by serum sodium concentration levels which reflect the composition of the fluids retained. Each type of overhydration presents different pathophysiologic effects. There are three types of overhydration:

- Isotonic overhydration
- Hypertonic overhydration
- Hypotonic overhydration

Overhydration or edema is commonly seen in patients with congestive heart failure, low blood pressure, renal insufficiency, liver failure (ascites) and physical inactivity. The fluid retention is usually a symptom of a bigger medical problem.

Edema is usually treated with loop diuretics. Overdose of loop diuretics can cause extracellular fluid depletion and a potassium deficiency. The success of loop diuretics is measured by a significant weight loss and a decrease in edema. Laboratory tests will change rapidly as edema diminishes. Typical lab values seen in edema are summarized in Table 5. Additional information about each laboratory test is in the next section of this text.

TABLE 5. SCREENING FOR OVERHYDRATION

Lab Test	Hypotonic	Isotonic	Hypertonic
Osmolality (S)	< normal	WNL	> normal
Sodium, (S)	< normal	WNL	> normal
Albumin (S)	< normal	WNL or slightly low	< normal
H/H	< normal	WNL or slightly low	< normal
BUN	< normal	WNL or slightly low	< normal

Key: WNL= within normal limits

ASSESSMENT OF PROTEIN STATUS

Assessment of protein status is essential for baseline assessment and to predict risk for malnutrition and skin failure. A patient's protein status is a reflection of the body's ability to synthesize dispensable amino acids (DAA) and to absorb and utilize indispensable amino acids (IAA). As the protein status declines the patient is at higher risk for infection, delayed wound healing and new skin breakdown. The traditional method to estimate visceral protein status is using a variety of lab test results including retinol binding protein level, prealbumin (transthyretin) and serum albumin. However all of these measures are negative acute phase proteins and are dramatically affected by inflammatory processes. Changes in these values do not appear to reflect changes in nutritional status. For more information refer to Protein, Blood, for more information on retinol binding protein, prealbumin and albumin.

NITROGEN BALANCE STUDIES

Nitrogen balance studies reflect the balance between exogenous nitrogen intake (by mouth or parenteral) and renal removal of nitrogen containing compounds (urinary, fecal, wound and other nitrogen sources). Nitrogen balance studies are often part of research studies to determine if the endogenous protein is being utilized. However, in a healthcare setting, nitrogen balance studies are not a measure of protein anabolism and catabolism because true protein turnover studies require consumption of labeled (stable isotope) protein to track protein utilization (Hoffenberg, 1966). The acutely ill patient is losing protein rapidly due to the inflammatory process, traumatic or surgical wounds. In addition, it is unclear if increasing exogenous protein will ameliorate the loss of endogenous protein. Adequate nutrition and specifically high biological value protein cannot circumvent the inflammatory metabolism, but may prevent excessive loss of muscle mass and immunosuppression (Griffiths, 1996).

Nitrogen balance studies are challenging to achieve because valid 24-hour urine collections are difficult to obtain unless the patient has a catheter. In addition, changes in renal function are common in patients with inflammatory metabolism, making standard nitrogen balance calculations inaccurate without calculation of nitrogen retention. In these patients, urea kinetics provides a more accurate estimation of nitrogen balance.

URINARY CREATININE

Creatinine is formed from creatine, a compound found almost exclusively in muscle tissue. Creatine is synthesized from the amino acids glycine and arginine with addition of a methyl group. It is a high-energy phosphate buffer, maintaining a constant supply of ATP for muscle contraction. Creatinine has no specific biologic function. It is continuously released from the muscle cells and excreted by the kidneys with little reabsorption. When a patient follows a meat-restricted diet, the size of the patient's somatic (muscle) protein pool is directly proportional to the amount of creatinine excreted. The clinical significance is that men generally excrete larger amounts of creatinine than women do and that individuals with greater muscular development excrete larger amounts than those who are less muscular. Total body weight is not proportional to creatinine excretion. Creatinine excretion rate is related to muscle mass in healthy individuals.

The use of urinary creatinine to assess somatic protein status in a healthcare setting in which patients are consuming a mixed diet has its limitations. Creatine is a component of muscle meats which is converted to creatinine. The body can not distinguish between the two sources of creatinine. In addition, urinary creatinine can vary significantly within individuals, probably due to sweat losses. Urinary creatinine concentration as a biomarker of muscle mass is typically used only in research.

NUTRITIONAL ANEMIAS

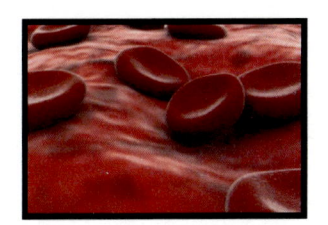

Anemia is symptomatic of a disease and is a biomarker for increased morbidity, mortality, hospitalizations and healthcare costs. It is a significant clinical finding and efforts should be made to determine its etiology (Andrews, 1999; Rockey, 1999).

The prevalence of anemia increases with each decade of life over age 70 and is associated with both frailty and mobility impairment (AMDA, 2007). Macrocytic anemia in older adults is often due to insufficient dietary vitamin B12 or folic acid. Other causes of macrocytic anemia include kidney disease, hemolytic anemia, hypothyroidism, or certain medications.

With aging, there is a decrease in iron in RBC (Fischbach, 2008; Corbett, 2000). The mechanism is not known, although iron seems to be absorbed from the intestine. However, there is a decreased incorporation of iron into the RBC resulting in lower hemoglobin levels (Beers, 2005). The significance of this drop in hemoglobin is not known. In addition, MCV (MCV) increases slightly with age.

Anemia is a deficiency in the erythrocyte mass and hemoglobin contents. A low hemoglobin or hematocrit needs to be evaluated further by a complete blood cell count (CBC), including hemoglobin concentration, hematocrit, red blood cell mass, and MCV (Blackwell, 2001). Norms are assuming adequate hydration. If the patient is dehydrated, the values will be falsely high. Overhydration will result in falsely low values.

Patients with an infection or other inflammatory processes present often have low hemoglobins and hematocrits related to redistribution of iron rather than a change in nutritional status. With infection, the cytokine interleukin-1β (IL-1β) inhibits the production and release of transferrin while stimulating the synthesis of ferritin. The net result is that iron is moved from transferrin and hemoglobin to ferritin. The redistribution of iron stores is a protective mechanism since many virulent bacterium have specialized receptors for iron uptake. The survival of the bacterium within the host is dependent upon its ability to extract nutrients from the surrounding environment.

CLASSIFICATION OF ANEMIAS

Anemias are classified by etiology. The causes include:
- Blood loss
- Deficient erythropoiesis
- Excessive hemolysis

BLOOD LOSS

Anemias can result from acute or chronic blood loss. Identification of the cause of the blood loss and resolution of the loss will most likely resolve the anemia. The lost erythrocyte mass and hemoglobin content will be replaced via transfusion or erythropoiesis (Blackwell, 2001).

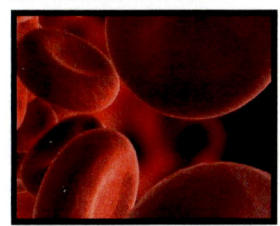

DEFICIENT ERYTHROPOIESIS

Anemias due to a deficient erythropoiesis include microcytic anemias, normochromic-normocytic anemias and macrocytic anemias. All of these anemias are characterized by low hemoglobins and hematocrits (Blackwell, 2001). The distinction is made by examining the MCV (Coulter, 1991). This test provides the average size of the patient's red blood cell. In microcytic anemias the heme or globin synthesis is deficient or defective resulting in a lower than normal MCV. In normocytic anemia the bone marrow failure prevents the erythroid mass from expanding as needed, but the volume is normal, so the MCV is normal. Megaloblastic erythropoiesis results when DNA or RNA synthesis is impaired. The MCV then exceeds normal values (Blackwell, 2001). Other tests used to evaluate erythropoiesis include reticulocyte count, red blood cell count, erythrocyte count and red blood cell width (RDW).

EXCESSIVE HEMOLYSIS

Anemia due to destruction of RBC is much less common and rarely associated with blood loss or bone marrow failure. These anemias are caused by defects that are either extrinsic or intrinsic to the RBC. For example, an anemia with extrinsic defects is autoimmune hemolysis. An anemia with intrinsic defects is sickle cell disease.

CATEGORIES OF NUTRITIONAL ANEMIAS

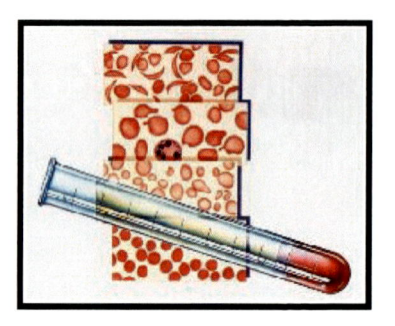

There are 4 categories of anemias and 4 types of nutritional anemias. Early onset of all of the nutritional anemias are associated with lack of energy, malaise and decreased interest in activities of daily living and lifelong interests. However, each presents a different pattern of laboratory results from a variety of blood tests. More than one type of nutritional anemia can occur at the same time. No one test alone is used to diagnose the nutritional anemias. Because the nutritional anemias can initially appear to be the same, it is important to look at more than one lab test result before recommending a plan for medical nutrition therapy.

Nutritional anemias are categorized using red blood cell indices quantifying the size, weight and hemoglobin concentration of red blood cells. These tests are used to categorize anemias. Table 6 categorizes nutritional anemias by red blood cell indices. The four types of nutritional anemias are:

- Iron Deficiency Anemia
- Megaloblastic Anemia
- Pernicious Anemia
- Anemia of Chronic and Inflammatory Diseases

IRON DEFICIENCY ANEMIA

Iron deficiency anemia is most commonly seen in children with low iron intakes. However, approximately 20 percent of women, 50 percent of pregnant women, and 3 percent of men are iron deficient. The DRI for iron for adult males and females 51 years and older is 8 mg/d. For females under the age of 50, the DRI is 18 mg/d. The NHANES data reports that median intakes of iron for adults aged 40 to 59 and 60 years and older are 15.5 mg/day and 14.8 mg/d respectively (Ervin, 2004).

Iron deficiency anemia may be the result of a chronic blood loss, after an acute blood loss, deficient diet, malabsorption of iron or increased need for iron. Decreased stomach acidity, due to overconsumption of antacids, ingestion of alkaline clay, achlorhydria, partial gastrectomy or weight loss surgery may lead to impaired iron absorption and ultimately iron deficiency anemia.

Clinical signs and symptoms include inflammation of the tongue, lips or mucous membranes of the mouth and spooned nails. In its advanced state, it is described as a microcytic hypochromic anemia. Laboratory tests used to diagnose iron deficiency anemia include a low hemoglobin, low hematocrit, low MCV, low serum iron, elevated total iron binding capacity (TIBC), low reticulocyte count, low ferritin, elevated RDW and elevated erythrocyte sedimentation rate. Not all of these tests may be available due to cost restraint. The MCV is the key test to examine once a low hemoglobin and low hematocrit are identified.

Once underlying causes of iron deficiency anemia are identified and addressed, oral iron therapy is preferred, however a multivitamin may be better tolerated. Absorption is best on an empty stomach, but may cause gastric upset (Blackwell, 2001). Remember that the goal of pharmacological intervention is to increase the deficient body components while avoiding a negative impact on the total dietary intake of the patient.

ANEMIA OF CHRONIC AND INFLAMMATORY DISEASES

Anemia of chronic and inflammatory diseases develops as a result of an extended infection or inflammation. The anemia usually manifests itself in a similar manner to iron deficiency anemia. While the physical signs and symptoms are the same as iron deficiency, anemia of chronic and inflammatory diseases is a normochromic-normocytic anemia. In anemia of chronic and inflammatory diseases, the lab results are below normal ranges for hemoglobin, hematocrit, serum iron and TIBC. However, the MCV and ferritin are usually normal. The changes in lab test

TABLE 6. ANEMIAS ACCORDING TO RBC INDICES

Normocytic[1], Normochromic[2], Anemia
■ Iron Deficiency (early stages)
■ Anemia of Chronic and Inflammatory Diseases
■ Acute Blood Loss
■ Pernicious Anemia (about 40% of cases)
Microcytic[3], Hypochromic[4] Anemia
■ Iron Deficiency (advanced)
Microcytic[3] Normochromic[1] Anemia
■ Renal Disease due to loss of erythropoietin
Macrocytic[5], Normochromic[1] Anemia
■ Vitamin B12 / Pernicious Anemia
■ Folic Acid Deficiency/Megaloblastic Anemia

Key: [1] Normocytic - normal RBC size
  [2] Normochromic - normal color (normal hemoglobin content)
  [3] Microcytic - smaller than normal RBC size
  [4] Hypochromic - less than normal color (↓ hemoglobin content)
  [5] Macrocytic - larger than normal RBC size

results are either related to redistribution of iron stores or impaired utilization. A multivitamin supplement with iron or oral iron therapy may be ordered, however, should be carefully monitored for expected outcomes. In cases of true anemia of chronic and inflammatory diseases, the lab values will not improve until the underlying condition resolves.

Other characteristics of anemia of chronic and inflammatory diseases may include slow involuntary weight loss and hypoalbuminemia. Weight loss occurs despite efforts to increase caloric intake. Certain chronic infections and inflammatory diseases cause several changes in the blood cell production system. These include a slightly shortened red blood cell life span and an isolation of iron in inflammatory cells (macrophages) that result in a decrease in the amount of iron available to make RBC. In the presence of these effects, a low-to-moderate grade anemia develops.

Conditions associated with the anemia of chronic and inflammatory diseases include the following:

- Advanced age
- AIDS
- Chronic Bacterial Endocarditis
- Chronic Renal Failure
- Congestive Heart Failure
- Crohn's Disease
- Juvenile Rheumatoid Arthritis
- Osteomyelitis
- Rheumatic fever
- Ulcerative Colitis

MACROCYTIC ANEMIAS

Macrocytic anemias include megaloblastic anemia or folate deficiency and pernicious anemia or vitamin B12 deficiency. The presence of macrocytic RBC requires evaluation of both folate and vitamin B12 status.

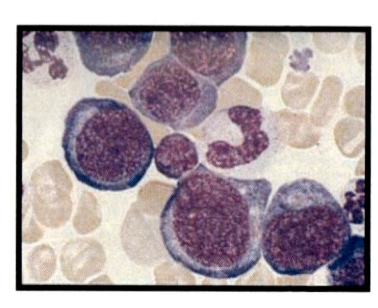

The metabolic interrelationship between folate and vitamin B12 may explain why a single deficiency of either leads to the same hematological changes. The most common cause of macrocytic anemia is megaloblastic anemia due to impaired DNA synthesis. Vitamin B12 and folate coenzymes are required for thymidylate and purine synthesis. A deficiency of either or both nutrients retards DNA synthesis that triggers dyspoiesis (abnormal rate of RBC maturation in bone marrow) and pancytopenia (decrease in the production of RBC). While the macrocytic RBC is the hallmark of macrocytic anemia, other rapidly dividing cells are affected. Other physiological changes may include, sore tongue due to glossitis or atrophy of tongue, skin changes, and flattening of intestinal villi (Guyton, 2006).

RNA synthesis is unaffected by a deficiency of folate or vitamin B12 but, there is a build up of cytoplasmic components in a slowly dividing cell making the RBC larger than normal. The primary defect in DNA synthesis caused by folate or vitamin B12 deficiency is a depletion of thymidine triphosphate (dTTP). This leads to retarded mitosis and nuclear maturation. The RBC have shortened life spans and reduced capacity to carry hemoglobin. Iron is stored as serum iron or ferritin rather than in hemoglobin (Guyton, 2006).

The first sign of inadequate folic acid intake is a decrease in serum folate concentration followed by a decrease in erythrocyte folate concentration and a rise in homocysteine levels. When folate supply to the bone marrow becomes rate limiting for erythropoiesis, macrocytic cells are produced. Macrocytic anemia is not evident in the early stages of folate deficiency because of the 120-day lifespan of normal erythrocytes.

When dietary vitamin B12 is deficient, the body cannot convert N^{5}methyl THF to the active form of folate, tetrahydrofolate

(THF). Without adequate vitamin B12, folate is trapped in an unusable form (Guyton, 2006). When dietary folate is deficient, the same problems occur because there are inadequate amounts of THF needed for the cascade of reactions required for DNA synthesis (Guyton, 2006). A B12 deficiency will eventually cause a folate deficiency because folate cannot be converted into an active form without vitamin B12 (Bostom, 1996).

One of the earliest clinical signs of both folate and vitamin B_{12} deficiency is hyper-segmentation of > 5 percent of neutrophils. Hyper-segmentation may also occur in uremia, myeloproliferative disorders, myelofibrosis and as a congenital lesion in 1% of the population. More testing is required to differentiate between megaloblastic and pernicious anemia.

The abnormal RBC cannot conform to the size of small capillaries. Instead, they fracture and hemolyze, thus shortening their lifespan. The macrocytic RBC has a reduced capacity to carry hemoglobin. Dietary iron is absorbed by the body and stored as serum iron or ferritin rather than in hemoglobin. Once the folate and/or vitamin B12 deficiency is treated through dietary supplements, the iron stores from the serum iron and ferritin will shift back to the RBC and the hemoglobin and hematocrit will return to normal levels. Homocysteine levels may or may not return to normal levels with folate supplementation.

MEGALOBLASTIC ANEMIA

Megaloblastic anemia is a folate deficiency commonly seen in middle-aged and older adults. It has been associated with an increased risk for heart disease and end stage renal disease because of the association with elevated homocysteine levels (Morrison, 1996; Pancharuniti, 1994; Robinson, 1996). It may be due to increased needs, a deficient diet, malabsorption of folate and/or a vitamin B12 deficiency. Malabsorption of folic acid may occur in individuals with diseases of the small intestine including ileitis, tropical and nontropical sprue, overgrowth of bacteria, hemolytic anemia, liver disease, malnutrition and following biliopancreatic diversion with and without duodenal switch (BPD/DS) weight loss surgery (Aills, 2008).

Some medications are folate antagonists and interfere with nucleic acid synthesis. The most common folate antagonists are anticonvulsants, antimalarials, alcohol, aminopterin and methotrexate. Megaloblastic anemia occurs after approximately 5 months of folate depletion.

The initial clinical signs and symptoms of megaloblastic anemia are low levels of hemoglobin, hematocrit and red cell folate. However, elevated levels of serum iron, MCV, ferritin and homocysteine are common. Falsely elevated concentrations of red cell folate are seen in patients with raised reticulocyte counts and low levels occur in vitamin B12 deficiency. Plasma folate can be used to assess status however; it is affected by recent folate intake.

Treatment for megaloblastic anemia is based on its etiology. Folate supplementation of 1 mg or more daily can compensate for vitamin B12 deficiency in DNA synthesis reversing macrocytic anemia and thereby masking vitamin B12 deficiency. Undiagnosed vitamin B12 deficiency will result in progressive permanent neurological damage including permanent changes in cognitive abilities. Individuals taking known folic acid antagonists will require prescription strength supplemental folate for as long as these medications are taken. Individuals with malabsorption disorders due to disease or weight loss surgery will require supplemental folic acid for a lifetime.

PERNICIOUS ANEMIA

Pernicious anemia is due to a vitamin B12 deficiency commonly seen in older adults, vegetarians and individuals who have had malabsorptive weight loss surgery. Early signs and symptoms include pallor, weakness, lightheadedness, smooth, sore tongue, diarrhea alternating with constipation, numbness and tingling of extremities, gait abnormalities, personality changes, irritability, confusion, cognitive changes, depression and numbness of the hands and feet. Permanent nerve lining damage and significant cognitive decline will result from an untreated vitamin B12 deficiency.

Absorption and utilization of vitamin B12 is a multi step process. Dietary vitamin B12 is bound to a protein carrier. An acidic environment is required for the body to cleave the protein carrier from vitamin B12. Once vitamin B12 is released from its protein carrier in the stomach, it must form a complex with intrinsic factor (IF) for absorption in the terminal ileum. IF is synthesized in the stomach in the presence of an acidic environment. Without IF, B12 cannot be absorbed, body stores are depleted and the body produces enlarged immature RBC. It is categorized as a macrocytic normochromic anemia, however about

40 percent of the cases are normocytic (Allen, 1990; Carmel, 1996; Koepke, 1997; Pennypacker, 1992).

The ability to absorb and utilize vitamin B12 decreases with age affecting about 20-50 percent of the elderly. The decline in absorption and utilization of vitamin B12 is primarily due to atrophic gastritis and/or gastric mucosa defect resulting in inadequate secretion of IF. Atrophic gastritis results in declining gastric acid and pepsinogen secretions. The increased pH in the gastrointestinal tract decreases intestinal absorption of the cobalamin protein complexes from food. In addition, the reduced acid secretion leads to an alkalinization of the small intestine, which may result in bacterial overgrowth and further decrease the bioavailability of the vitamin.

Other causes of pernicious anemia include history of gastric or ileal resections, weight loss surgery, diseases associated with malabsorption (e.g. Crohn's disease) may cause impaired vitamin B12 absorption. Medications such as proton pump inhibitors or H2 receptor antagonists inhibit the intestinal absorption of vitamin B12.

Plasma vitamin B12 test is a reflection of recent intake rather than vitamin stores. More prolonged vitamin B12 deficiency is measured by either blood or urinary methylmalonic acid (MMA). Elevated serum and urinary MMA levels are direct measure of tissue vitamin B12 activity. Urinary MMA/creatinine ratio is more accurate than the serum MMA as it indicates tissue/cellular vitamin B12 deficiency.

The etiology of vitamin B12 deficiency should be determined for appropriate treatment. Vitamin B12 deficiency can result from either inadequate diet or impaired absorption.

The Schilling test can be used to distinguish insufficient secretion of intrinsic factor from malabsorption syndromes. In this test, radioactive B12 is taken orally and urinary excretion is measured over 24 hours. A flushing dose of unlabeled B12 is given with the labeled B12 to saturate liver storage and enhance labeled B12 excretion.

Normally, >7 percent of the labeled B12 is recovered in the urine. If absorption is low, it is necessary to repeat the test with administration of intrinsic factor. The lab results for pernicious anemia are very similar to megaloblastic anemia. Lower than normal values are seen for hemoglobin, hematocrit and serum B12. However, elevated levels are seen in serum iron, serum folate, ferritin and homocysteine. MCV may be elevated or normal. The only definitive lab test appears to be MMA. This test is elevated in vitamin B12 deficiency and normal in megaloblastic anemia (Van Asselt, 1996; Savage, 1994).

Treatment for pernicious anemia is based on the etiology of the anemia. Oral B12 supplements are effective if the body can produce adequate levels of IF and the pH of the stomach is sufficient to cleave vitamin B12 from its protein carrier. However, if the body is unable to produce IF then daily B12 nasal spray, B12 patch or monthly injections of B12 are recommended. Table 7 summarizes the most commonly used tests to evaluate for different types of anemia. Not all patients' lab results will follow the pattern provided in Table 7 due to the effects of other diseases or the use of medications. Additional information about each laboratory test is included in the next section of this text.

TABLE 7. GUIDE TO ANEMIAS

Lab Test	Fe Deficiency	Megaloblastic Anemia (Folate)	Pernicious Anemia (B_{12})	Anemia of Chronic & Inflammatory Disease
HGB Females Males	<12 gm <14 gm	<12 gm <14 gm	<12 gm <14 gm	<12 gm <14 gm
HCT Females Males	<37% <42%	<37% <42%	<37% <42%	<37% <42%
MCV	<80 µm³	>95 µm³	>95 µm³ or WNL	WNL
MCH	<27 pg	>31 pg	>31 pg	WNL
Serum Fe Females Males	<60 µg/dL <80 µg/dL	>190 µg/dL >180 µg/dL	>190 µg/dL >180 µg/dL	<60 µg/dL <80 µg/dL
TIBC	>460 µg/dL	-	-	<250 µg/dL
Retic Count	> 2%	< 0.5%	< 0.5%	< 0.5%
ESR	elevated	elevated	elevated	elevated
Ferritin Females	<10 ng/mL	>150 ng/mL	>150 ng/mL	WNL or elevated
Ferritin Males	<12 ng/mL	>300 ng/mL	>300 ng/mL	WNL or elevated
Serum B_{12}	normal	decreased	decreased	WNL
Folate	-	<5 ng/mL	>25 ng/mL	WNL or decreased
Hcy	-	increased	increased	WNL
MMA	-	WNL	increased	-

KEY:
HGB=hemoglobin, HCT=hematocrit, MCV=mean corpuscular volume, MCH= mean corpuscular hemoglobin, TIBC=total iron binding capacity, Retic count= reticulocyte count, ESR= erythrocyte sedimentation rate, Hcy=homocysteine, MMA= methylmalonic acid

REVIEW QUESTIONS FOR CRITICAL THINKING

1. What do laboratory tests tell the healthcare practitioner about the patient's health status?

2. What questions should the health practitioner ask himself/herself before requesting laboratory tests?

3. Why might there be a difference in the reference standards used in this text and the standards used in a healthcare institution?

4. Describe how the hydration status of a patient impacts the interpretation of the lab results. Include dehydration and overhydration.

5. Identify the key labs used to diagnose dehydration and overhydration.

6. Describe the relationship between inflammatory response and acute phase proteins.

7. Identify the ranges in all four types of anemias. Explain how to differentiate between the different nutritional anemias.

ALANINE AMINOTRANSFERASE (ALT)
(formerly called SGPT)

NORMAL VALUES
Infants: May be twice as high as adult normal ranges
Adult/child: 4 - 36 U/L at 37°C; 4 - 36 U/L (SI)
Elderly: slightly higher than adults
Values may be higher in men and in African Americans

NUTRITIONAL SIGNIFICANCE

Alanine aminotransferase (ALT) is an enzyme found primarily in the liver and to a lesser degree in the kidneys, heart and skeletal muscle. Injury to the liver results in elevated levels.

In hepatitis, values may be 8 to 20 times normal values during the prodromal and clinical phases. Lactic dehydrogenase (LDH) and aspartate aminotransferase (AST) are also elevated. Serum AST levels are often compared with ALT. The AST:ALT ratio > 1.0 is seen in alcoholic cirrhosis, liver congestion and metastatic tumor of the liver. The AST:ALT ratio < 1.0 is seen in acute hepatitis, viral hepatitis and infectious mononucleosis.

RELATED TESTS: AST, GGTP, ALP, CK, LDH

Increased with:
- Cholestasis
- Hepatocellular disease
  - hepatitis
  - hepatic ischemia
  - cirrhosis or necrosis
  - tumor
- Hepatotoxic drugs
- Infectious mononucleosis
- Myocardial infarction

Decreased with:
- Malnutrition
- Urinary tract infection

Alanine Aminotransferase (ALT) (formerly called SGPT)

Increased with:
- Myositis
- Obstructive jaundice
- Pancreatitis
- Severe burns
- Shock
- Trauma to striated muscle

Medications that may increase levels:

Abacavir	Acarbose	Adefovir
Acebutolol	Acetaminophen	Acetohexamide
Acyclovir	Albendazole	Aldesleukin
Allopurinol	Alprazolam	Aminoglutethimide
Aminosalicylic acid	Amiodarone	Amitriptyline
Amoxapine	Amphotericin B	Ampicillin
Amrinone	Anabolic steroids	Anastrazole
Anticonvulsants	Antifungal agents	Ardeparin
Aprepitant	Aripiprazole	Atomoxetine
Arsenic trioxide	Asparaginase	Atorvastatin
Atovaquone	Auranofin	Aurothioglucose
Azathioprine	Azithromycin	Aztreonam
Barbiturates	Barium	BCG vaccine
Benazepril	Bepridil	Betaxolol
Bicalutamide	Bismuth subsalicylate	Bisoprolol
Bitolterol	Bromocriptine	Bupropion
Busulfan	Calcitriol	Candesartan
Capecitabine	Carbamazepine	Carbenicillin
Carmustine	Cephalosporin	Cerivastatin
Cetirizine	Chenodiol	Chlorambucil
Chloramphenicol	Chlordiazepoxide	Chlorothiazide
Chlorpheniramine	Chlorpromazine	Chlorpropamide
Chlortetracycline	Chlorthalidone	Chloral hydrate
Chlorzoxazone	Cholestyramine	Choline magnesium trisalicylate
Cidofovir	Cimetidine	Cinoxacin
Ciprofloxacin	Cisplatin	Cladribine
Clarithromycin	Clindamycin	Clofazimine
Clofarabine	Clomipramine	Colchicine
Clofibrate	Clomiphene	Clonidine

ALANINE AMINOTRANSFERASE (ALT)
(formerly called SGPT)

Medications that may increase levels:

Clopidogrel	Clorazepate	Cloxacillin
Clozapine	Codeine	Colestipol
Cortisone	Cyclobenzaprine	Cyclophosphamide
Cyproheptadine	Cytarabine	Dactinomycin
Dalteparin	Danazol	Dantrolene
Dapsone	Demeclocycline	Desipramine
Diazepam	Diclofenac	Dicumarol
Diazoxide	Eletriptan	Eplerenone
Didanosine	Dienestrol	Diethylstilbestrol
Diflunisal	Diltiazem	Disopyramide
Disulfiram	Docetaxel	Doxorubicin
Doxycycline	Dronabinol	Enalapril
Enoxacin	Enoxaparin	Erythromycin
Erlotinib	Fosinopril	Furosemide
Estrogens	Dacarbazine	Desmopressin
Estropipate	Ethacrynic acid	Ethambutol
Ethchlorvynol	Ether	Etodolac
Etoposide	Etretinate	Famotidine
Felbamate	Fenofibrate	Fenoprofen
Flecainide	Fluconazole	Flucytosine
Fluorouracil	Fluoxymesterone	Fluphenazine
Flurazepam	Flutamide	Fluvastatin
Fluvoxamine	Foscarnet	Fosphenytoin
Furazolidone	Ganciclovir	Gamma globulin
Garlic	Gemcitabine	Gemfibrozil
Gentamicin	Glimepiride	Glyburide
Glycopyrrolate	Gold	Goserelin
Granisetron	Griseofulvin	Guanethidine
Haloperidol	Heparin	Hepatitis A vaccine
Hepatitis B vaccine	Hydralazine	Hydrochlorothiazide
Hydroflumethiazide	Ibuprofen	Idarubicin
Imatinib	Imipenem/cilastin	Imipramine
Indinavir	Indomethacin	INH
Interferon	Interleukin	Infliximab
Iron	Isosorbide dinitrate	Isotretinoin
Isradipine	Ifosfamide	Itraconazole
Kanamycin	Ketamine	Ketoconazole
Ketoprofen	Ketorolac	Labetalol
Lamotrigine	Lansoprazole	Leflunomide
Levamisole	Levodopa	

ALANINE AMINOTRANSFERASE (ALT)
(formerly called SGPT)

Medications that may increase levels:

Levothyroxine
LMW heparins
Loratadine
Loxapine
Medroxyprogesterone
Melphalan
Mercaptopurine
Metaxalone
Methotrexate
Methylphenidate
Methyltestosterone
Metoprolol
Mirtazapine
Moexipril
Moricizine
Muromonab-CD3
Nalidixic acid
Naproxen
Nelfinavir
Nevirapine
Nicardipine
Nitazoxanide
Nitrofurantoin
Norfloxacin
Ofloxacin
Omeprazole
Oxacillin
Oxymetholone
Pargyline
Pemoline
Pentoxifylline
Phenelzine
Phenylbutazone
Pindolol
Piroxicam
Pravastatin
Procainamide
Propoxyphene
Pyrazinamide

Lincomycin
Lomefloxacin
Losartan
MAO inhibitors
Mechlorethamine
Mefenamic acid
Meperidine
Meropenem
Methenamine
Methoxsalen
Metoclopramide
Mexiletine
Mitomycin
Molindone
Morphine
Mycophenolate
Naltrexone
Nafarelin
Nefazodone
Niacinamide
Nilutamide
Nifedipine
Nizatidine
Nortriptyline
Oleandomycin
Ondansetron
Oxaprozin
Palivizumab
Paroxetine
Penicillamine
Perphenazine
Phenobarbital
Phenytoin
Pioglitazone
Polythiazide
Prazosin
Prochlorperazine
Propranolol
Pyrimethamine

Lisinopril
Loracarbef
Lovastatin
Maprotiline
Meclofenamate
Mefloquine
Meprobamate
Mesalamine
Methimazole
Methyldopa
Metolazone
Minocycline
Mitoxantrone
Montelukast
Moxalactam
Nabumetone
Nandrolone
Nafcillin
Netilmicin
Niacin
Nisoldipine
Nitisinone
Norethandrolone
Octreotide
Olsalazine
Oral contraceptives
Oxazepam
Papaverine
Pegaspargase
Pentamidine
Phenazopyridine
Phenothiazine
Phosphorus
Piperacillin
Pralidoxime
Probenecid
Propafenone
Propylthiouracil
Quazepam

ALANINE AMINOTRANSFERASE (ALT) (formerly called SGPT)

Medications that may increase levels:

Quinapril	Quinidine	Ramipril
Ranitidine	Riluzole	Risperidone
Ritonavir	Rosiglitazone	Rifampin
Saquinavir	Sargramostim	Semustine
Sibutramine	Sildenafil	Simvastatin
Sodium oxybate	Sparfloxacin	Spectinomycin
Stanozolol	Stavudine	Streptokinase
Streptomycin	Streptozocin	Sulfadiazine
Sulfamethoxazole	Sulfanilamide	Sulfasalazine
Sulfisoxazole	Sulfonylureas	Sulindac
Sumatriptan	Tacrine	Tacrolimus
Tadalafil	Tamoxifen	Tegaserod
Terbinafine	Terbutaline	Tetracycline
Thiabendazole	Thiazides	Thiethylperazine
Thiocyanate	Thioguanine	Thiopental
Thioridazine	Thiothixene	Thiouracil
Ticarcillin	Ticlopidine	Timolol
Tinzaparin	Tobramycin	Tocainide
Tolazamide	Tolazoline	Tolbutamide
Tolcapone	Tolmetin	Topotecan
Tramadol	Trandolapril	Tranylcypromine
Trastuzumab	Tretinoin	Triazolam
Trichlormethiazide	Trifluoperazine	Trimethoprim
Trimetrexate	Trimipramine	Trioxsalen
Triptorelin	Troglitazone	Troleandomycin
Trovafloxacin	Uracil mustard	Ursodiol
Valproic acid	Valsartan	Venlafaxine
Verapamil	Vidarabine	Vitamin A
Vitamin C	Warfarin	Zalcitabine
Zidovudine	Zileuton	Zolmitriptan
Zolpidem		

Medications that may decrease levels:

Aspirin	Carvedilol	Cyclosporine
Interferon	Ketoprofen	Phenothiazine
Simvastatin	Toremifene	Ursodiol

ALKALINE PHOSPHATASE (ALP)

NORMAL VALUES
Child/Adolescent:
    < 2 yr: 85-235 U/L; 1.4-3.9 µKat/L(SI)
    2-8 yrs: 65-210 U/L; 1.08-3.5 µKat/L(SI)
    9-15 yr: 60-300 U/L; 1.0-5.0 µKat/L(SI)
    16-21 y:r   30-200 U/L; 0.5-3.3 µKat/L(SI)
Adults: 30-120 U/L; 0.5-2.0 µKat/L(SI)
Elderly: slightly higher than adults

NUTRITIONAL SIGNIFICANCE

Alkaline phosphatase (ALP) is an enzyme found primarily in the bone, liver and biliary tract. One unique feature of this phosphatase enzyme is its function is increased in an alkaline environment. Recent ingestion of a meal can increase ALP levels. The presence of ALP suggests a variety of liver and bone disorders including metastatic tumors to the liver.

ALP is normally elevated during the third trimester of pregnancy, in growing children and adolescents because of bone growth. In bone disease, ALP levels rise in proportion to new bone cell production and deposits of calcium in bones. In liver disease, the serum levels rise when excretion of this enzyme is impaired due to obstruction in the biliary tract.

Isoenzymes of ALP are used to distinguish between liver and bone diseases. ALP1 is from the liver and ALP2 is from the bone. The isoenzyme of liver origin is heat stable while the isoenzyme of bone origin is inactivated by heat. Another test used to determine the source of elevated ALP is to simultaneously test for ALP and 5'-nucleotidase. The 5'-nucleotidase is primarily made

ALKALINE PHOSPHATASE (ALP)

by the liver. If total ALP and 5'-nucleotidase are both elevated the disease is most likely in the liver. However, if 5'-nucleotidase is normal and total ALP is elevated, the disease is likely in the bone.

RELATED TESTS: ALT, AST, GGT, 5'-nucleotidase, CK, LDH, LAP

Increased with:
- Amyloidosis
- Biliary cirrhosis
- Bone disease
- Healing bone fracture
- Cancer lung, pancreas
- Chronic alcohol ingestion
- Cytomegalovirus
- Diabetes mellitus
- Gilbert's syndrome
- Rickets
- Sarcoidosis
- Ulcerative colitis
- Hodgkin's disease
- Hyperparathyroidism
- Hyperphosphatasia
- Hyperthyroidism
- Infectious mononucleosis
- Intrahepatic or extrahepatic biliary obstruction
- Liver disease
  - hepatitis
  - hepatocellular cirrhosis
  - liver metastasis
- Metastatic bone cancer
- Normal growing children
- Normal pregnancy
- Obstructive jaundice
- Osteogenic sarcoma

Decreased with:
- Celiac disease
- Excess vitamin B ingestion
- Hypophosphatemia
- Hypothyroidism
- Magnesium deficiency
- Milk-alkali syndrome
- Malnutrition
- Pernicious anemia
- Scurvy
- Vitamin D excess
- Zinc deficiency

Alkaline Phosphatase (ALP)

Increased with:
- Osteomalacia
- Paget's disease
- Rheumatoid arthritis
- Intestinal ischemia or infarction

Medications that may increase levels:

Acebutolol	Acetaminophen	Acetohexamide
Acyclovir	Albendazole	Aldesleukin
Allopurinol	Alprazolam	Aminoglutethimide
Aminosalicylic acid	Amiodarone	Amitriptyline
Amoxapine	Amphotericin B	Ampicillin
Amrinone	Anabolic steroids	Anastrazole
Anticonvulsants	Antifungal agents	Ardeparin
Arsenic trioxide	Asparaginase	Atorvastatin
Atovaquone	Auranofin	Aurothioglucose
Azathioprine	Azithromycin	Aztreonam
Barbiturates	Barium	BCG vaccine
Benazepril	Bepridil	Betaxolol
Bitolterol	Bromocriptine	Bupropion
Busulfan	Calcitriol	Candesartan
Capecitabine	Carbamazepine	Carbenicillin
Carmustine	Capreomycin	Captopril
Carvedilol	Cephalosporin antibiotics	Cerivastatin
Cetirizine	Chenodiol	Chloramphenicol
Chlordiazepoxide	Chloroform	Chlorothiazide
Chlorpheniramine	Chlorpromazine	Chlorpropamide
Chlorzoxazone	Cidofovir	Cimetidine
Cinoxacin	Ciprofloxacin	Clindamycin
Clofibrate	Clonidine	Clozapine
Colchicine	Colestipol	Conjugated estrogens
Cyclobenzaprine	Cyclophosphamide	Cycloserine
Cyclosporine	Cyproheptadine	Cytarabine
Dactinomycin	Danazol	Dantrolene
Dapsone	Demeclocycline	Desipramine
Diazepam	Diazoxide	Diclofenac
Didanosine	Diltiazem	Disopyramide
Disulfiram	Docetaxel	Doxorubicin
Doxycycline	Enalapril	Erythromycin

Alkaline Phosphatase (ALP)

Medications that may increase levels:

Estropipate	Ethacrynic acid	Ethambutol
Ether	Ethionamide	Etretinate
Famotidine	Felodipine	Fenoprofen
Flecainide	Fluconazole	Flucytosine
Fluorouracil	Fluoxymesterone	Fluphenazine
Flurazepam	Flutamide	Fluvastatin
Foscarnet	Fosphenytoin	Ganciclovir
Gemcitabine	Gemfibrozil	Gentamicin
Glimepiride	Glyburide	Glycopyrrolate
Griseofulvin	Guanethidine	Haloperidol
Hepatitis A vaccine	Hepatitis B vaccine	HGF
Hydralazine	Hydroflumethiazide	Ibuprofen
Idarubicin	Ifosfamide	Imipenem/cilastin
Imipramine	Indomethacin	INH
Interferon	Interleukin	Irinotecan
Isradipine	Itraconazole	Kanamycin
Ketamine	Ketoconazole	Ketoprofen
Ketorolac	Labetalol	Lamotrigine
Lansoprazole	Leflunomide	Levodopa
Levothyroxine	Lincomycin	Lisinopril
Lithium	Lomefloxacin	Loracarbef
Loratadine	Lovastatin	MAO inhibitors
Mechlorethamine	Meclofenamate	Medroxyprogesterone
Melphalan	Meprobamate	Mercaptopurine
Meropenem	Mesalamine	Metaxalone
Methimazole	Methotrexate	Methoxsalen
Methyldopa	Methyltestosterone	Metoclopramide
Metolazone	Metoprolol	Minocycline
Mirtazapine	Misoprostol	Mitoxantrone
Moexipril	Molindone	Morphine
Moxalactam	Mycophenolate	Nabumetone
Nafarelin	Nalidixic acid	Naltrexone
Nandrolone	Naproxen	Nelfinavir
Netilmicin	Niacin	Niacinamide
Nicardipine	Nifedipine	Nilutamide
Nitrofurantoin	Nizatidine	Norethandrolone
Norfloxacin	Nortriptyline	Octreotide
Ofloxacin	Oleandomycin	Olsalazine
Omeprazole	Oxacillin	Oxaprozin
Oxazepam	Oxymetholone	Papaverine
Pargyline	Paroxetine	

Alkaline Phosphatase (ALP)

Medications that may increase levels:

Pegaspargase	Penicillamine	Perphenazine
Phenazopyridine	Phenobarbital	Phenothiazine
Phenytoin	Phosphorus	Pindolol
Piperacillin	Piroxicam	Polythiazide
Probenecid	Procainamide	Prochlorperazine
Promazine	Promethazine	Propafenone
Propoxyphene	Propylthiouracil	Protriptyline
Pyrazinamide	Pyrimethamine	Quazepam
Quinapril	Quinethazone	Quinidine
Ramipril	Ranitidine	Rifampin
Riluzole	Risperidone	Sargramostim
Sildenafil	Spectinomycin	Stanozolol
Streptokinase	Sulfadiazine	Sulfamethoxazole
Sulfanilamide	Sulfasalazine	Sulfisoxazole
Sulfonylureas	Sulindac	Tacrolimus
Terbinafine	Tetracycline	Thiabendazole
Thiazides	Thiethylperazine	Thioguanine
Thiopental	Thioridazine	Thiothixene
Thiouracil	Ticarcillin	Ticlopidine
Timolol	Tocainide	Tolazamide
Tolazoline	Tolbutamide	Tolcapone
Tolmetin	Toremifene	Tramadol
Trastuzumab	Tretinoin	Triazolam
Trichlormethiazide	Trifluoperazine	Trimethoprim
Trimetrexate	Trimipramine	Trioxsalen
Troglitazone	Troleandomycin	Trovafloxacin
Uracil mustard	Ursodiol	Valproic acid
Venlafaxine	Verapamil	Vidarabine
Vitamin D	Warfarin	Zalcitabine
Zidovudine	Zolmitriptan	Zolpidem

Medications that may decrease levels:

Acyclovir	Alendronate	Aluminum antacids
Antithyroid therapy	Arsenicals	Azathioprine
Calcitonin	Calcitriol	Carvedilol
Chemotherapy	Clofibrate	Colchicine
Cyanides	Cyclosporine	Danazol
Estrogens	Etidronate	Norethindrone
Oral contraceptives	Oxalates	Pamidronate
Prednisone	Tamoxifen	Trifluoperazine
Ursodiol	Zinc salts	

AMMONIA, BLOOD

NORMAL VALUES
Newborn: 90-150 mcg/dL; 53-88 µmol/L (SI)
Child: 40-80 mcg/dL; 23-47 µmol/L (SI)
Adults: 10-80 mcg/dL; 6-47 µmol/L (SI)

NUTRITIONAL SIGNIFICANCE

Ammonia is a by-product of protein metabolism. Most of the ammonia is synthesized in the gut by bacteria. The liver converts it into urea for excretion. Elevated serum levels are seen in severe liver dysfunction and when the blood flow to the liver is altered as in portal hypertension. In both cases, the ammonia cannot be converted to urea and ammonia levels rise. Elevated levels of ammonia affect the body's acid-base balance and brain function. Reduction of ammonia levels is essential.

The blood levels of ammonia are primarily used in the diagnosis and follow up of hepatic encephalopathy, Reye's syndrome and hepatic coma. In chronic liver disease, a specific event such as gastrointestinal bleeding, excessive protein intake, diuretics, paracentesis, hypokalemia, acute infections, surgery, azotemia or administration of morphine or ammonia containing medications may trigger hepatic encephalopathy. When laboratory evaluation is not available, observation of clinical features of hepatic encephalopathy are used for diagnosis. Cigarette smoking can produce significant increases in ammonia levels.

When renal status is impaired, ammonia levels can rise due to the kidney's inability to excrete ammonia. The elevated

AMMONIA, BLOOD

levels due to renal impairment can also result in encephalopathy and coma. Reference standards for ammonia vary based on the test methodology used. Arterial ammonia levels are more reliable than venous levels, but are more difficult to obtain.

RELATED TESTS: ALT, AST, ALP

Increased with:
- Asparagine intoxication
- GI bleeding
- GI obstruction
- GI infection
- Genetic metabolic disorder of urea cycle
- Hemolytic disease of the newborn
- Hepatic disease
  - coma
  - encephalopathy
- HHH syndrome
  - hyperornithinemia
  - hyperammonemia
  - hypocitrullinuria
- Parenteral nutrition
- Portal hypertension
- Pulmonary emphysema
- Renal failure
- Reye's syndrome
- Severe heart failure with congestive hepatomegaly
- Ureterosigmoidostomy

Decreased with:
- Essential hypertension
- Malignant hypertension

Medications that may increase levels:

Acetazolamide	Alcohol	Ammonia chloride
Asparaginase	Barbiturates	Chlorothiazide
Chlorthalidone	Ethacrynic acid	Felbamate
Furosemide	Hydroflumethiazide	INH

AMMONIA, BLOOD

Medications that may increase levels:
Ion exchange resins   Pegaspargase   Tetracycline
Thiazides   Valproic acid

Medications that may decrease levels:
Cefixime   Cefotaxime   Diphenhydramine
Kanamycin   Lactobacillus   lactulose
                  acidophilus
Levodopa   MAO Inhibitors   Neomycin
Potassium salts   Tetracycline   Tromethamine

APOLIPOPROTEIN A & B, (Apo A-I, Apo B, Apo A-I/ Apo B ratio), LIPOPROTEIN (a [LP(a)], APOLIPOPROTEIN E (APO E)

NORMAL VALUES
APO A-I
Newborn Males:	41-93 mg/dL; 0.41-0.93 g/L (SI)
Newborn Females:	38-106 mg/dL; 0.38-1.06 g/L (SI)
6 mos-4 yr Males:	67-167 mg/dL; 0.67-1.67 g/L (SI)
6 mos-4 yr Females:	60-148 mg/dL; 0.6-1.48 g/L (SI)
5 yr -17 yr:	83-115 mg/dL; 0.83-1.51 g/L (SI)
Adult/Elderly Males:	75-160 mg/dL; 0.75-1.6 g/L (SI)
Adult/Elderly Females:	80-175 mg/dL; 0.80-1.75 g/L (SI)

APO B
Newborn:	11-31 mg/dL; 0.11-0.31 g/L (SI)
6 mos- 3 yr:	23-75 mg/dL ; 0.23-0.75 g/L (SI)
5 yr -17 yr Male:	47-139 mg/dL ; 0.47-1.39 g/L (SI)
5 yr -17 yr Female:	41-132 mg/dL ; 0.41-1.32 g/L (SI)
Adult/Elderly Males:	50-125 mg/dL; 0.50-1.25 g/L (SI)
Adult/Elderly Females:	45-120 mg/dL; 0.45-1.20 g/L (SI)

APO A-I/ APO B RATIO
Males:	0.8-2.24
Females:	0.76-3.23

LIPOPROTEIN (a)
Caucasian (5th to 95th percentile)
Males:	2.2- 49.4 mg/dL ; 0.22-0.49 g/L (SI)
Females:	2.1- 57.3 mg/dL; 0.21- 0.57 g/L (SI)

African-American (5th to 95th percentile)
Males:	4.6-71.8 mg/dL ; 0.46-0.72 g/L (SI)
Females:	4.4-75 mg/dL; 0.44-0.75 g/L (SI)

NUTRITIONAL SIGNIFICANCE

Apo A-I constitutes about 75 percent of apo A in HDL. Apo A-II constitutes about 20 percent of the total HDL protein. As a general rule, as HDL levels increases, so do apo A levels.

APOLIPOPROTEIN A & B, (Apo A-I, Apo B, Apo A-I/ Apo B ratio), LIPOPROTEIN (a [LP(a)], APOLIPOPROTEIN E (APO E)

Physical exercise may increase apo A-I levels. Eating a diet high in carbohydrates and polyunsaturated fats and smoking may decrease apo A-I levels. Some experts have proposed that apo A is a better index of risk for atherosclerosis than HDL assay.

Apo B is the major polypeptide component of LDL and VLDL. Approximately 80 percent of the protein in LDL is apo B and about 40 percent of the protein in VLDL is apo B. Apo B has two main forms apo B-48 and apo B-100. Apo B-100 is synthesized in the liver and found in lipoproteins of endogenous origin. It is the principal transport mechanism for endogenous cholesterol. Apo B-100 has an affinity for the LDL receptor sites located on the cell surfaces of peripheral tissues. It is involved in deposition of cholesterol in tissues. Eating a diet that is high in saturated fats and cholesterol may increase apo-B levels. Some experts propose that apo B-100 may be a better index for risk of atherosclerosis than LDL assay. Apo B-48 is synthesized in the intestines and is mainly found in chylomicrons. It serves as a carrier for ingested lipids through the intestines into the blood stream. Diets high in saturated fats and cholesterol may increase apo B levels. Some experts have proposed that apo B is a better indicator of risk for atherosclerosis than LDL.

Decreased levels of apo A and increased levels of apo B-100 are associated with increased risk of coronary heart disease. A low ratio of apo A to apo B may also be a risk factor.

APOLIPOPROTEIN A & B, (Apo A-I, Apo B, Apo A-I/ Apo B ratio), LIPOPROTEIN (a [LP(a)], APOLIPOPROTEIN E (APO E)

Lp(a) or 'lipoprotein little a' is another lipoprotein particle found in LDL. It is similar in chemical structure to plasminogen. Some experts believe that Lp(a) is a mutation of plasminogen. Plasminogen is the precursor of the proteolytic enzyme plasmin. This enzyme is responsible for dissolving fibrin clots. It has been proposed that Lp(a) is an independent risk factor for atherosclerosis because of its relationship to plasminogen. Microthrombi containing fibrin on the vessel walls become incorporated into the arthrosclerotic plaque. Some researchers propose that following endothelial damage, Lp(a) may become incorporated into the arterial wall, inhibiting the cleavage of fibrin in microthrombi by competing with plasminogen for access to fibrin. Atherosclerotic damage of the arterial wall occurs and results in occlusive disease or an aneurysm. Familial hypercholesterolemia, some forms of renal failure, nephrotic syndrome and estrogen depletion in women over the age of 50 have been associated with increased levels of Lp(a). Individuals with increased levels of Lp(a) appear to have a much higher risk for coronary heart disease.

All of the lipoproteins are acute phase reactants and can be elevated in acutely and chronically ill patients. Levels fall when inflammatory processes wane.

Apo E is involved in the transport of cholesterol. It has three alleles: E-2, E-3 and E-4. The apo E-4 gene has been

APOLIPOPROTEIN A & B, (Apo A-I, Apo B, Apo A-I/ Apo B ratio), LIPOPROTEIN (a [LP(a)], APOLIPOPROTEIN E (APO E)

proposed as a risk factor for Alzheimer's disease. While apo E-4 allele has a strong association with Alzheimer's disease, it is unclear how the apo E functions as a risk factor for modifying the age of onset of Alzheimer's disease. Apo E is present in neuritic amyloid plaques and may be involved in neurotic tangle formations since it binds with tau proteins.

RELATED TESTS: LDL-C, HDL-C

Apo A-I Increased with:
- Familial hyperalphalipoproteinemia
- Pregnancy
- Weight reduction

Apo A-I Decreased with:
- Familial hypoalphalipoproteinemia
- Ischemic coronary disease
- Myocardial infarction
- Coronary heart disease
- Uncontrolled diabetes mellitus
- Tangier's disease
- Nephrotic syndrome
- Chronic renal failure
- Cholestasis
- Hemodialysis
- Fish eye disease
- Hepatocellular disease
- Familial hypertriglyceridemia

Medications that may increase Apo-A-I:

Carbamazepine	Estrogens	Ethanol
Furosemide	Gemfibrozil	Lovastatin
Niacin	Nisoldipine	Oral contraceptives
Phenobarbital	Phenytoin	Pravastatin
Prednisolone	Simvastatin	

Medications that may decrease Apo-A-I:
Lovastatin

Apolipoprotein A & B, (Apo A-I, Apo B, Apo A-I/ Apo B ratio), Lipoprotein (a [Lp(a)], Apolipoprotein E (Apo E)

Apo B Increased with:
- Hyperlipoproteinemia (types IIa, IIb, IV, V)
- Nephrotic syndrome
- Pregnancy
- Hemodialysis
- Biliary obstruction
- Coronary artery disease
- Diabetes mellitus
- Hypothyroidism
- Anorexia nervosa
- Hepatic disease & obstruction
- Porphyria
- Cushing's syndrome
- Werner's syndrome

Apo B Decreased with:
- Hyperlipoproteinemia (type I)
- Hyperthyroidism
- Malnutrition
- Inflammatory joint disease
- Chronic pulmonary disease
- Weight reduction
- Chronic anemia
- Reye's syndrome
- Tangier's disease
- Apo C-II deficiency

Medications that may increase Apo B:

Androgens	Beta blockers	Diuretics
Ethanol abuse	Progestins	Amiodarone
Atenolol	Chlorthalidone	Estrogen
Cyclosporine	Progestin	Etretinate
Furosemide	Gemfibrozil	Isotretinoin
Levonorgestrel	Methyclothiazide	Metoprolol
Oral contraceptives	Phenobarbital	Radioactive iodine
Simvastatin	Stanozolol	

Medications that may decrease Apo B:

Atorvastatin	Bisoprolol	Captopril
Cholestyramine	Colestipol	Doxazosin
Estrogen	Fenofibrate	Gemfibrozil
Indomethacin	Interferon alfa-2a	Interferon beta-1b
Ketoconazole	Levothyroxine	Lisinopril
LMW hepatins	Losartan	Lovastatin
Neomycin	Niacin	Nicotinic acid
Nifedipine	Phenytoin	Pravastatin
Prazosin	Prednisolone	Probucol
Psyllium	Raloxifene	Simvastatin
Tacrolimus	Thyroxine	

APOLIPOPROTEIN A & B, (Apo A-I, Apo B, Apo A-I/ Apo B ratio), LIPOPROTEIN (a [LP(a)], APOLIPOPROTEIN E (APO E)

Lp(a) Increased with:
- Premature CAD
- Stenosis of cerebral arteries
- Uncontrolled DM
- Severe hypothyroidism
- Familial hypercholesterolemia
- Chronic renal failure
- Estrogen depletion

Lp(a) Decreased with:
- Alcoholism
- Malnutrition
- Chronic liver disease

Medications that may decrease Lp(a):
Estrogens   Niacin   Neomycin
Stanozolol

Apo E Increased with:
- Alzheimer's disease
- Type III hyperlipoproteinemia

ARTERIAL BLOOD GASES (ABGs) (pH, BICARBONATE (HCO3), CARBON DIOXIDE (CO2), PCO2, PO2, O2 SATURATION)

NORMAL VALUES

pH
Newborn:	7.32-7.49
2 mos- 2yr:	7.34-7.46
Adult/Child:	7.35-7.45

CARBON DIOXIDE (CO_2)
Newborn:	13-122 mEq/L; 13-122 mmol/L (SI)
Infant/Child:	20-28 mEq/L; 20-28 mmol/L (SI)
Adults/Elderly:	23 - 30 mEq/L; 23 - 30 mmol/L(SI)

PCO_2
Child < 2 yr:	26-41 mm Hg
Adult/Child:	35-45 mm Hg

BICARBONATE HCO_3
Newborn/Infant:	16-24 mEq/L; 16-24 mmol/L
Adult/Child:	21-28 mEq/L; 21-28 mmol/L

PO_2
Newborn:	60-70 mm Hg
Adult/Child:	80-100 mm Hg

O_2 SATURATION
Newborn:	40-90%
Adult/Child:	95-100%
Elderly:	95%

NUTRITIONAL SIGNIFICANCE

Measurement of arterial blood gasses (ABGs) provides data to assess and manage a patient's respiratory and metabolic acid/base and electrolyte homeostasis. It is also used to evaluate adequacy of oxygenation.

Arterial Blood Gases (ABGs) (pH, Bicarbonate (HCO3), Carbon Dioxide (CO2), PCO2, PO2, O2 Saturation)

pH

The pH of any fluid is the measure of the hydrogen ion (H-) concentration. A pH of 7 is neutral. The pH is inversely proportional to the actual hydrogen ion concentration. The lower the pH, the more acidic the blood and the higher the pH, the more alkaline the blood is. In metabolic alkalosis is pH > 7.4 and acidity pH < 7.35. In respiratory or metabolic alkalosis the pH is elevated and in respiratory or metabolic acidosis, the pH is decreased. See Tables 8 and 9.

Bicarbonate (HCO3) & Carbon Dioxide (CO2)

The CO_2 content is a measure of levels in blood. It serves as a biomarker for the renal system, provides a means of assessing the acid-base status and is a tool to evaluate the electrolyte status. The CO_2 content measures the H_2CO_3 dissolved in CO_2 and in the serum. Since the amounts of H_2CO_3 and dissolved CO_2 are minute amounts in the blood, the CO_2 content is an indirect measure of the HCO_3 anion. The HCO_3 anion is second in importance to the chloride ion in electrical and intracellular fluid. As the HCO_3 level increases the pH increases. HCO_3 is elevated in metabolic alkalosis and is low in metabolic acidosis. In metabolic acidosis, decreased levels are primarily caused by renal disease. Acidosis results from excess acid into the body fluid.

Alkalosis occurs due to excess loss of acid, producing chloride levels above the norms of 98 to 106 mmol/L. The body must cope with carbonic acid, which is derived from the hydration

Arterial Blood Gases (ABGs) (pH, Bicarbonate (HCO3), Carbon Dioxide (CO2), PCO2, PO2, O2 Saturation)

of CO2 and fixed hydrogen ions. The lungs remove the volatile CO2. Retention of CO2 results in acidosis. Excessive loss of CO2 results in alkalosis. The hydrogen ions are associated with organic and inorganic anions. These ions are buffered in body fluids. They can only be excreted by the kidneys or lost through other fluids via the GI tract. The values of BUN and creatinine are critical in evaluating the CO2 levels or acid-base balance.

In diabetic acidosis, the supply of ketoacids exceeds the demands of the cell. Blood plasma acids rise and plasma HCO3 decreases because it is used to neutralize these excess acids. A patient in shock will have a build up of lactic acid that is buffered by the HCO3. Plasma levels will diminish to neutralize these excess acids. The patient with COPD will have increased HCO3 to compensate for the chronic hypoventilation (i.e. compensation respiratory acidosis). CO2 level and pH are inversely proportional. As the CO2 level increases the pH decrease.

PCO2

CO2 test is often confused with PCO_2 ; a measure of the partial pressure of CO2 in the blood. PCO_2 reflects ventilation capacity because it is the major stimulant to the breathing center of the brain. A patient who is breathing very deeply and very fast is blowing off more CO2, and PCO_2 levels drop. If PCO2 levels rise too high, breathing cannot keep up with the demand to blow off

ARTERIAL BLOOD GASES (ABGs) (pH, BICARBONATE (HCO3), CARBON DIOXIDE (CO2), PCO2, PO2, O2 SATURATION)

CO2. Ultimately, the brain and ventilation are depressed, resulting in coma. The PCO_2 level is elevated in primary respiratory acidosis and decreased in primary respiratory alkalosis.

TABLE 8. ABG with Acid-Base Disturbances

Acid-Base Disturbance	pH	PCO2 (mm Hg)	HCO3 (mEq/L)
Normal Values	7.35-7.45	35-45	22-26
Respiratory acidosis	↓	↑	WNL
Respiratory alkalosis	↑	↓	WNL
Metabolic acidosis	↓	WNL	↓
Metabolic alkalosis	↑	WNL	↑

TABLE 9. Compensatory Responses in Acid-Base Disturbances

Acid-Base Disturbance	Mode of Compensation
Respiratory acidosis	Kidneys retain ↑ HCO3 → ↑ pH
Respiratory alkalosis	Kidneys excrete ↑ HCO3 → ↓ pH
Metabolic acidosis	Lungs blow off CO2 → ↑ pH
Metabolic alkalosis	Lungs retain CO2 → ↓ pH

PO2

PO2 is an indirect measure of the oxygen content of arterial blood measuring the tension or pressure of oxygen dissolved in the plasma. The pressure determines the force of O2 to diffuse across the pulmonary alveoli membrane.

O2 SATURATION

Oxygen saturation is a ratio between the actual O2 content

ARTERIAL BLOOD GASES (ABGs) (pH, BICARBONATE (HCO3), CARBON DIOXIDE (CO2), PCO2, PO2, O2 SATURATION)

of hemoglobin and the potential maximum O_2 carrying capacity. The percentage indicates the relationship between hemoglobin and O_2. It does not indicate the O_2 content of the blood. The maximum amount of O_2 that can be combined with hemoglobin is called the oxygen capacity. The combined measurements of oxygen saturation, PO_2 and hemoglobin indicate the amount of O_2 available to the tissues, is called 'sats.'

As the PCO_2 level decreases, the percentage of hemoglobin saturation also decreases. When the PCO_2 drops below 60 mm Hg, small decreases in the PO_2 cause large decreases in the percentage of hemoglobin saturation with O_2. At O_2 saturation of 70 percent or lower, the tissues are unable to extract enough O_2 to carry out vital functions.

RELATED TESTS: BUN, creatinine, hemoglobin

pH Increased with:
Metabolic alkalosis
- hypokalemia
- hypochloremia
- chronic high volume gastric suction
- Na HCO3 administration
- aspirin intoxication
- aldosteronism
- chronic vomiting

pH Decreased with:
Metabolic acidosis
- ketoacidosis
- lactic acidosis
- severe diarrhea
- strenuous exercise
- renal failure

pH Increased with:
Respiratory alkalosis
- chronic heart failure
- cystic fibrosis
- shock

pH Decreased with:
Respiratory acidosis
- respiratory failure
- neuromuscular depression
- ventilatory failure

ARTERIAL BLOOD GASES (ABGs) (pH, BICARBONATE (HCO3), CARBON DIOXIDE(CO2), PCO2, PO2, O2 SATURATION)

pH Increased with:
Respiratory alkalosis
- pulmonary emboli
- CO poisoning
- pulmonary diseases
- anxiety neuroses
- pain
- pregnancy
- myocardial infarction
- CNS diseases
- anemia

pH Decreased with:
Respiratory acidosis
- obesity
- pulmonary edema
- cardiopulmonary arrest

Medications that may increase pH levels:
Mercurial diuretics   Steroids(megadose)

CO2 Increased with:
- Severe vomiting
- Aldosteronism
- High volume gastric suction
- Emphysema
- COPD
- Metabolic alkalosis
- Chronic use of mercurial diuretics

CO2 Decreased with:
- Severe diarrhea
- Starvation
- Renal failure
- Diabetic ketoacidosis
- Shock
- Metabolic acidosis
- Chronic use of chlorothiazide diuretics
- Salicylate toxicity

Medications that may increase CO2 levels:
Aldosterone	Barbiturates	Bicarbonates
Ethacrynic acid	Hydrocortisone	Loop diuretics
Mercurial diuretics	Steroids	

Medications that may decrease CO2 levels:
Methicillin	Nitrofurantoin	Paraldehyde
Phenformin hydrochloride	Tetracycline	Thiazide diuretics
Triamterene		

Arterial Blood Gases (ABGs) (pH, Bicarbonate (HCO3), Carbon Dioxide(CO2), PCO2, PO2, O2 Saturation)

HCO3 Increased with:
- Aldosteronism
- High volume gastric suction
- Chronic vomiting
- COPD

HCO3 Decreased with:
- Starvation
- Chronic use of loop diuretics
- Acute renal failure
- Diabetic ketoacidosis
- Metabolic acidosis
- Salicylate toxicity
- Chronic & severe diarrhea

PCO2 Increased with:
- COPD
- Bronchitis
- Emphysema
- Oversedation
- Head trauma
- Over oxygenation in COPD patient
- Pickwickian syndrome

PCO2 Decreased with:
- Hypoxemia
- Pulmonary emboli
- Anxiety
- Pain
- Pregnancy

PO2 & O2 Increased with:
- Polycythemia
- Increased inspired O2
- Hyperventilation

PO2 & O2 Decreased with:
- Anemias
- Mucus plug
- Bronchospasm
- Atelectasis
- Pneumothorax
- Pulmonary edema
- ARDS
- Restrictive lung disease
- Cardiac septal defects
- Emboli
- Inadequate inspired O2 (suffocation)
- Severe hypoventilation
  - oversedation
    - neurologic somnolence

Aspartate Aminotransferase (AST) (formerly SGOT)

Normal Values

Newborn 0-5 days:	35-140 IU/L; 0.58- 2.34 µKat/L (SI)
< 3 yr:	15-60 IU/L; 0.25- 1.0 µKat/L (SI)
3-6 yr:	15-50 IU/L; 0.25- 0.84 µKat/L (SI)
6-12 yr:	10-50 IU/L; 0.17- 0.84 µKat/L (SI)
12-18 yr:	10-40 IU/L; 0.17- 0.67 µKat/L (SI)
Adults/child:	0-35 IU/L; 0-.58 µKat/L (SI)
Elderly:	slightly higher than adults

Nutritional Significance

AST is an enzyme primarily found in the heart, liver, skeletal muscle cells and to a lesser degree in the kidneys and pancreas. It is used as a diagnostic tool when coronary occlusive heart disease or hepatocellular disease is suspected. AST enzyme is tested in the cardiac enzyme series along with troponin T, creatine kinase (CK) and lactic dehydrogenase (LDH).

When disease or injury damage cells the AST is released into the blood. The rise in AST is directly related to the number of cells affected by the disease or injury. Typically, AST levels rise about 8 hours after cell injury. With a myocardial infarction (MI), AST levels rise within 6 to 10 hours, peak between 12 to 48 hours and return to normal in 3 to 7 days unless more cardiac injury occurs. AST levels are monitored to estimate the time of the MI. If the AST begins to rise a second time, this suggests that there is more cardiac injury despite therapy. The levels do not rise in angina, pericarditis or rheumatic carditis.

When damage to the liver occurs, there is an elevated AST level. If the damage is acute, the levels rise, peak at up to 20 times

ASPARTATE AMINOTRANSFERASE (AST) (formerly SGOT)

the normal value, then fall. The elevation is directly related to the degree of active inflammation. However, if the injury is chronic, the elevated levels persist. Serum AST levels are often compared with alanine aminotransferase (ALT). The AST:ALT ratio > 1.0 is seen in alcoholic cirrhosis, liver congestion and metastatic tumor of the liver. The AST:ALT ratio < 1.0 is seen in acute hepatitis, viral hepatitis and infectious mononucleosis. The ratio is less accurate if the AST level exceeds 10 times the norm.

RELATED TESTS : CK, ALT, LDH, LAP, GGTP, ALP, 5'-nucleotidase.

Increased with:
- Acute renal failure
- Biliary obstruction
- Cardiac diseases:
  - angioplasty
  - cardiac surgery
  - cardiac catheterization
  - congestive heart failure
  - cerebral infarction
  - myocardial infarction
- Convulsions
- Dermatomyositis
- Gangrene
- Hemolytic anemia, acute
- Hypothyroidism
- Mononucleosis
- Mushroom poisoning
- Pancreatitis, acute
- Pulmonary emboli

Decreased with:
- Azotemia
- Vitamin B6 deficiency
- Beriberi (thiamin deficiency)
- Diabetic ketoacidosis
- Kidney disorders
  - acute renal disease
  - renal dialysis
  - uremia
- Liver disease, chronic
- Pregnancy

ASPARTATE AMINOTRANSFERASE (AST) (formerly SGOT)

Increased with:
- Hepatic diseases:
  - hepatitis
  - hepatic cirrhosis
  - necrosis
  - drug-induced liver injury
  - hepatic metastasis
  - hepatic surgery
  - infectious mononucleosis with hepatitis
- Reye's syndrome
- Skeletal Muscle Diseases
  - skeletal muscle trauma
  - burns
  - progressive muscular dystrophy
  - heat stroke
  - polymyositis
  - myopathy
- Toxic shock syndrome
- Recent non-cardiac surgery

Medications that may increase levels:

Abacavir	Acarbose	Adefovir
Acebutolol	Acetaminophen	Acetohexamide
Acyclovir	Albendazole	Aldesleukin
Allopurinol	Alprazolam	Aminoglutethimide
Aminosalicylic acid	Amiodarone	Amitriptyline
Amoxapine	Amphotericin B	Ampicillin
Amrinone	Anabolic steroids	Anastrazole
Anticonvulsants	Antifungal agents	Ardeparin
Aprepitant	Aripiprazole	Atomoxetine
Arsenic trioxide	Asparaginase	Atorvastatin
Atovaquone	Auranofin	Aurothioglucose
Azathioprine	Azithromycin	Aztreonam
Barbiturates	Barium	BCG vaccine

Aspartate Aminotransferase (AST) (formerly SGOT)

Medications that may increase levels:

Benazepril	Bepridil	Betaxolol
Bicalutamide	Bismuth subsalicylate	Bisoprolol
Bitolterol	Bromocriptine	Bupropion
Busulfan	Calcitriol	Candesartan
Capecitabine	Carbamazepine	Carbenicillin
Carmustine	Cephalosporin	Cerivastatin
Cetirizine	Chenodiol	Chloral hydrate
Chlorambucil	Chloramphenicol	Chlordiazepoxide
Chlorothiazide	Chlorpheniramine	Chlorpromazine
Chlorpropamide	Chlortetracycline	Chlorthalidone
Chlorzoxazone	Cholestyramine	Choline magnesium trisalicylate
Cidofovir	Cimetidine	Cinoxacin
Ciprofloxacin	Cisplatin	Cladribine
Clarithromycin	Clindamycin	Clofarabine
Clofazimine	Clofibrate	Clomiphene
Clomipramine	Clonidine	Clopidogrel
Clorazepate	Cloxacillin	Clozapine
Codeine	Colchicine	Colestipol
Cortisone	Cyclobenzaprine	Cyclophosphamide
Cyproheptadine	Cytarabine	Dacarbazine
Dactinomycin	Dalteparin	Danazol
Dantrolene	Dapsone	Demeclocycline
Desipramine	Desmopressin	Diazepam
Diazoxide	Diclofenac	Dicumarol
Didanosine	Dienestrol	Diethylstilbestrol
Diflunisal	Diltiazem	Disopyramide
Disulfiram	Docetaxel	Doxorubicin
Doxycycline	Dronabinol	Eletriptan
Enalapril	Enoxacin	Enoxaparin
Eplerenone	Erlotinib	Erythromycin
Estrogens	Estropipate	Ethacrynic acid
Ethambutol	Ethchlorvynol	Ether
Etodolac	Etoposide	Etretinate
Famotidine	Felbamate	Fenofibrate
Fenoprofen	Flecainide	Fluconazole
Flucytosine	Fluorouracil	Fluoxymesterone
Fluphenazine	Flurazepam	Flutamide
Fluvastatin	Fluvoxamine	Foscarnet
Fosinopril	Fosphenytoin	Furosemide

ASPARTATE AMINOTRANSFERASE (AST) (formerly SGOT)

Medications that may increase levels:

Furazolidone	Ganciclovir	Gemcitabine
Gamma globulin	Garlic	Glyburide
Gemfibrozil	Gentamicin	Glimepiride
Glycopyrrolate	Goserelin	Granisetron
Gold	Heparin	Infliximab
Griseofulvin	Guanethidine	Haloperidol
Hepatitis A vaccine	Hepatitis B vaccine	Hydralazine
Hydrochlorothiazide	Hydroflumethiazide	Ibuprofen
Idarubicin	Ifosfamide	Imatinib
Imipenem/cilastin	Imipramine	Indinavir
Indomethacin	INH	Interferon
Interleukin	Iron	Isosorbide dinitrate
Isotretinoin	Isradipine	Itraconazole
Kanamycin	Ketamine	Ketoconazole
Ketoprofen	Ketorolac	Labetalol
Lamotrigine	Lansoprazole	Leflunomide
Levamisole	Levodopa	Levothyroxine
Lincomycin	Lisinopril	LMW heparins
Lomefloxacin	Loracarbef	Loratadine
Losartan	Lovastatin	Loxapine
MAO inhibitors	Maprotiline	Medroxyprogesterone
Mechlorethamine	Meclofenamate	Melphalan
Mefenamic acid	Mefloquine	Mercaptopurine
Meperidine	Meprobamate	Metaxalone
Meropenem	Mesalamine	Methotrexate
Methenamine	Methimazole	Methylphenidate
Methoxsalen	Methyldopa	Methyltestosterone
Metoclopramide	Metolazone	Metoprolol
Mexiletine	Minocycline	Mirtazapine
Mitomycin	Mitoxantrone	Moexipril
Molindone	Montelukast	Moricizine
Morphine	Moxalactam	Muromonab-CD3
Mycophenolate	Nabumetone	Nalidixic acid
Naltrexone	Nandrolone	Naproxen
Nafarelin	Nafcillin	Nelfinavir
Nefazodone	Netilmicin	Nevirapine
Niacinamide	Niacin	Nicardipine
Nilutamide	Nisoldipine	Nitazoxanide
Nifedipine	Nitisinone	Nitrofurantoin
Nizatidine	Norethandrolone	Norfloxacin
Nortriptyline	Octreotide	

Aspartate Aminotransferase (AST) (formerly SGOT)

Medications that may increase levels:

Ofloxacin	Oleandomycin	Olsalazine
Omeprazole	Ondansetron	Oral contraceptives
Oxacillin	Oxaprozin	Oxazepam
Oxymetholone	Palivizumab	Papaverine
Pargyline	Paroxetine	Pegaspargase
Pemoline	Penicillamine	Pentamidine
Pentoxifylline	Perphenazine	Phenazopyridine
Phenelzine	Phenobarbital	Phenothiazine
Phenylbutazone	Phenytoin	Phosphorus
Pindolol	Pioglitazone	Piperacillin
Piroxicam	Polythiazide	Pralidoxime
Pravastatin	Prazosin	Probenecid
Procainamide	Prochlorperazine	Propafenone
Propoxyphene	Propranolol	Propylthiouracil
Pyrazinamide	Pyrimethamine	Quazepam
Quinapril	Quinidine	Ramipril
Ranitidine	Riluzole	Risperidone
Ritonavir	Rosiglitazone	Rifampin
Saquinavir	Sargramostim	Semustine
Sibutramine	Sildenafil	Simvastatin
Sodium oxybate	Sparfloxacin	Spectinomycin
Stanozolol	Stavudine	Streptokinase
Streptomycin	Streptozocin	Sulfadiazine
Sulfamethoxazole	Sulfanilamide	Sulfasalazine
Sulfisoxazole	Sulfonylureas	Sulindac
Sumatriptan	Tacrine	Tacrolimus
Tadalafil	Tamoxifen	Tegaserod
Terbinafine	Terbutaline	Tetracycline
Thiabendazole	Thiazides	Thiethylperazine
Thiocyanate	Thioguanine	Thiopental
Thioridazine	Thiothixene	Thiouracil
Ticarcillin	Ticlopidine	Timolol
Tinzaparin	Tobramycin	Tocainide
Tolazamide	Tolazoline	Tolbutamide
Tolcapone	Tolmetin	Topotecan
Tramadol	Trandolapril	Tranylcypromine
Trastuzumab	Tretinoin	Triazolam
Trichlormethiazide	Trifluoperazine	Trimethoprim
Trimetrexate	Trimipramine	Trioxsalen
Triptorelin	Troglitazone	Troleandomycin
Trovafloxacin	Uracil mustard	Ursodiol

ASPARTATE AMINOTRANSFERASE (AST) (formerly SGOT)

Medications that may increase levels:

Valproic acid	Valsartan	Venlafaxine
Verapamil	Vidarabine	Vitamin A
Vitamin C	Warfarin	Zalcitabine
Zidovudine	Zileuton	Zolmitriptan
Zolpidem		

Medications that may decrease levels:

Allopurinol	Ascorbic acid	Clomipramine
Cyclosporine	Eletriptan	Ibuprofen
Ketoprofen	Metronidazole	Naltrexone
Penicillamine	Pindolol	Prednisone
Progesterone	Rifampin	Simvastatin
Toremifene	Trifluoperazine	Ursodiol

BILIRUBIN, BLOOD & URINE

NORMAL SERUM VALUES
TOTAL BILIRUBIN
Newborn: 1.0-12.0 mg/dL: 17.1-205 μmol/L (SI)
Child/Adult/Elderly: 0.3-1.0 mg/dL; 5.1- 7.0 μmol/L (SI)

INDIRECT BILIRUBIN
Child/Adult/Elderly: 0.2-0.8 mg/dL; 3.4-12.0 μmol/L (SI)

DIRECT BILIRUBIN
Child/Adult/Elderly: 0.1-0.3 mg/dL; 1.7-5.1 μmol/L (SI)

CRITICAL VALUES: TOTAL BILIRUBIN
Newborn: > 15 mg/dL; 257 μmol/L (SI)
Adult: > 12 mg/dL, 205 μmol/L (SI)

BILIRUBIN, URINE
Adults: 0-0.2 mg/dL; 0-0.34 μmol /L (SI)

NUTRITIONAL SIGNIFICANCE

    Bilirubin is a constituent of bile. The total serum bilirubin represents both the conjugated or direct and unconjugated or indirect bilirubin. Normally the unconjugated bilirubin makes up 70-85 percent of the total bilirubin. The level of conjugated or unconjugated bilirubin above normal ranges indicates the likely medical condition.

    Metabolism of bilirubin begins in the reticuloendothelial system with the breakdown of RBC. The RBC release hemoglobin and it is broken down into heme and globin. Heme is broken down to form biliverdin, which is then converted to indirect or unconjugated bilirubin. The unconjugated bilirubin travels to the liver and is conjugated with glucuronide resulting in conjugated or

BILIRUBIN, BLOOD & URINE

direct bilirubin. The conjugated bilirubin is excreted from the liver into the intrahepatic canaliculi, the hepatic ducts, the common bile duct and finally the bowel.

Jaundice is a condition in which the total serum bilirubin exceeds 2.5 mg/dL. The skin and whites of the eyes have a yellowish color due to the high levels of bilirubin. Jaundice results from a defect in metabolism or excretion of bilirubin. The defect can occur at any stage of heme catabolism. Elevated levels of conjugated bilirubin can occur when the defect in bilirubin metabolism occurs in the liver after the glucuronide addition. A classic example of direct or conjugated hyperbilirubinemia occurs when a gallstone blocks the bile duct.

In jaundice, if the conjugated bilirubin represents more than 50 percent of the total it is likely due to gallstones, tumor, inflammation or scarring. This is called conjugated hyperbilirubinemia. Jaundice of the newborn occurs when the neonate's liver does not have enough conjugating enzymes. The result is high levels of unconjugated bilirubin passing through the blood brain barrier and deposited in the brain causing encephalopathy or kernicterus. Unconjugated bilirubinemia is diagnosed when less than 15 to 20 percent of the total bilirubin is conjugated. The levels of unconjugated bilirubin are likely due to accelerated erythrocyte hemolysis, hepatitis or drugs.

Bilirubin is not normally found in the urine. However, if serum levels are high enough, conjugated bilirubin may be

BILIRUBIN, BLOOD & URINE

excreted in the urine. Bilirubin in the urine suggests that the disease affects bilirubin metabolism after conjugation or defects in excretion. Testing for bilirubin is part of a routine urine analysis.

RELATED TESTS: conjugated bilirubin, unconjugated bilirubin, GGT, ALP, AST, LDH, 5'-nucleotidase

Conjugated (direct) Bilirubin Increased with:
- Dubin-Johnson syndrome
- Cholestasis from meds
- Bile duct obstruction from:
  - tumor
  - scarring
  - gallstones
  - inflammation
  - surgical trauma
- Liver metastasis
- Rotor's syndrome

Unconjugated (indirect) Bilirubin Increased with:
- Erythroblastosis fetalis
- Sepsis
- blood transfusion (large-volume)
- Liver diseases
  - cirrhosis
  - hepatitis
  - Gilbert's Syndrome
- Hemolytic jaundice
- Pernicious anemia
- Sickle cell anemia
- Transfusion reaction
- Crigler-Najjar syndrome
- Hemolytic anemia
- Resolution of large hematoma

Medications that may increase blood levels:

Acarbose	Acebutolol	Acetaminophen
Acetazolamide	Acetohexamide	Acetophenazine
Acyclovir	Albendazole	Aldesleukin
Allopurinol	Alprazolam	Amiloride
Aminoglutethimide	Aminosalicylic acid	Amiodarone
Amitriptyline	Amoxapine	Amphotericin
Amrinone	Amyl nitrate	Anabolic steroids
Anastrazole	Anticonvulsants	Antifungal agents
Antimalarials	Antipyretics	Ascorbic acid
Asparaginase	Aspirin	Atazanavir

BILIRUBIN, BLOOD & URINE

Medications that may increase blood levels:

Atomoxetine	Atorvastatin	Auranofin
Azathioprine	Azithromycin	Barbiturates
BCG vaccine	Benazepril	Benzthiazide
Bevacizumab	Bicalutamide	Bismuth subsalicylate
Bleomycin	Bupropion	Busulfan
Candesartan	Captopril	Carbamazepine
Carbenicillin	Carmustine	Carvedilol
Cefazolin	Cefdinir	Cefoperazone
Cefoxitin	Cefpodoxime	Ceftazidime
Ceftibuten	Ceftizoxime	Ceftriaxone
Cefuroxime	Cephalothin	Cerivastatin
Cetirizine	Chenodiol	Chloral hydrate
Chlorambucil	Chloramphenicol	Chlordane
Chlordiazepoxide	Chloroform	Chloroquine
Chlorothiazide	Chlorpromazine	Chlorpropamide
Chlortetracycline	Chlorzoxazone	Cidofovir
Cimetidine	Cisplatin	Cladribine
Clindamycin	Clofarabine	Clofazimine
Clofibrate	Clonidine	Clopidogrel
Clozapine	Colchicine	Conjugated estrogens
Coumadin	Cyclobenzaprine	Cyclophosphamide
Cycloserine	Cyclosporine	Cyproheptadine
Cytarabine	Dacarbazine	Dactinomycin
Dantrolene	Dapsone	Desipramine
Dextrothyroxine	Diazepam	Diazoxide
Diclofenac	Dicloxacillin	Didanosine
Dienestrol	Diethylstilbestrol	Diflunisal
Diltiazem	Dimercaprol	Diphenhydramine
Disopyramide	Disulfiram	Docetaxel
Doxepin	Doxorubicin	Doxycycline
Duloxetine	Enalapril	Enoxaparin
Epinephrine	Erlotinib	Erythromycin
Escitalopram	Estramustine	Estropipate
Ethacrynic acid	Ethambutol	Ether
Ethionamide	Ethosuximide	Etoposide
Etretinate	Factor IX	Famotidine
Felbamate	Fenofibrate	Fenoprofen
Fluconazole	Flucytosine	Fluorouracil
Fluoxymesterone	Fluphenazine	Flurazepam
Flutamide	Fluvastatin	Fluvoxamin
Fosinopril	Fosphenytoin	Furazolidone

BILIRUBIN, BLOOD & URINE

Medications that may increase blood levels:

Furosemide	Ganciclovir	Gemcitabine
Gemfibrozil	Gentamicin	Glimepiride
Glyburide	Glycopyrrolate	Gold
Griseofulvin	Guanethidine	Haloperidol
Halothane	Hepatitis A vaccine	Hepatitis B vaccine
Hydralazine	Hydrochlorothiazide	Hydroflumethiazide
Hydroxyurea	Ibuprofen	Idarubicin
Imipramine	Indapamide	Indinavir
Indomethacin	Interferon	Interleukin
Irinotecan	Iron	Iron dextran
Isoniazid	Isotretinoin	Isradipine
Itraconazole	Kanamycin	Ketoconazole
Ketoprofen	Ketorolac	Labetalol
Lamivudine	Lamotrigine	Lansoprazole
Laronidase	Levamisole	Levodopa
Lincomycin	Lisinopril	Lomefloxacin
Losartan	Lovastatin	Loxapine
Lugol's iodine	MAO inhibitors	Medroxyprogesterone
Mefenamic acid	Melphalan	Meperidine
Meprobamate	Mercaptopurine	Meropenem
Mesalamine	Mesoridazine	Metaxalone
Methacholine	Methimazole	Methotrexate
Methoxsalen	Methsuximide	Methyclothiazide
Methyldopa	Methylene blue	Methylphenidate
Methyltestosterone	Metoclopramide	Metolazone
Minocycline	Mirtazapine	Mitomycin
Mitoxantrone	Molindone	Moricizine
Morphine	Moxalactam	Nabumetone
Nalidixic acid	Naproxen	Netilmicin
Nevirapine	Niacin	Niacinamide
Nicardipine	Nicotinic acid	Nitrofurantoin
Nitrofurazone	Nizatidine	Norethandrolone
Norethindrone	Nortriptyline	Novobiocin
Octreotide	Ofloxacin	Oleandomycin
Omeprazole	Oral contraceptives	Oxacillin
Oxaliplatin	Oxazepam	Oxymetholone
Papaverine	Pargyline	Paroxetine
Pegaspargase	Pemoline	Penicillamine
Penicillin	Pentoxifylline	Perphenazine
Phenazopyridine	Phenelzine	Phenobarbital
Phenothiazine	Phenytoin	Phosphorus

BILIRUBIN, BLOOD & URINE

Medications that may increase levels:

Piperacillin	Piroxicam	Polythiazide
Prazosin	Primaquine	Probenecid
Procainamide	Procarbazine	Prochlorperazine
Progesterone	Promazine	Promethazine
Propafenone	Propanolol	Propoxyphene
Propylthiouracil	Pyrazinamide	Quazepam
Quinapril	Quinethazone	Quinidine
Quinine	Quinupristin	Radiographic agents
Ramipril	Ranitidine	Reserpine
Rifampin	Riluzole	Salicylate
Saquinavir	Sargramostim	Sorbitan
Spironolactone	Stanozolol	Stavudine
Streptomycin	Sulfacetamide	Sulfadiazine
Sulfadoxine	Sulfamethizole	Sulfamethoxazole
Sulfasalazine	Sulfinpyrazone	Sulfisoxazole
Sulfonylureas	Sulindac	Tacrine
Tacrolimus	Tamoxifen	Telithromycin
Terbinafine	Testosterone	Tetracycline
Theophylline	Thiabendazole	Thiazides
Thiethylperazine	Thioguanine	Thiopental
Thioridazine	Thiothixene	Thiouracil
Ticarcillin	Ticlopidine	Timolol
Tobramycin	Tocainide	Tolazamide
Tolazoline	Tolbutamide	Tolcapone
Tolmetin	Topotecan	Toremifene
Tramadol	Trandolapril	Tranylcypromine
Trastuzumab	Tretinoin	Triazolam
Trichlormethiazide	Trifluoperazine	Trimethobenzamide
Trimethoprim	Trimetrexate	Trimipramine
Trioxsalen	Triptorelin	Troleandomycin
Uracil mustard	Ursodiol	Valproic acid
Venlafaxine	Verapamil	Vidarabine
Vinorelbine	Vitamin A	Vitamin K
Voriconazole	Warfarin	Zafirlukast
Zalcitabine	Zidovudine	Zinc
Ziprasidone	Zolmitriptan	Zolpidem

Medications that may decrease blood levels:

Amikacin	Anticonvulsants	Aspirin
Barbiturates	Caffeine	Carbamazepine
Cyclosporine	Hydroxyurea	Isotretinoin

BILIRUBIN, BLOOD & URINE

Medications that may decrease blood levels:
Penicillin	Pindolol	Prednisone
Sulfisoxazole	Theophylline	Thioridazine
Ursodiol	Valproic acid	

Urine Levels Increased with:
- Rotor's syndrome
- Gallstones
- Liver metastasis
- Bile duct obstruction from:
  - tumor
  - scarring
  - inflammation
  - surgical trauma
- Cholestasis from drugs
- Dubin-Johnson syndrome

Medications that may increase urine levels:
Acetohexamide	Acetophenazine	Allopurinol
Aminosalicylic acid	Antibiotics	Barbiturates
Chlorpromazine	Dapsone	Diuretics
Etodolac	Fluphenazine	Imipramine
Isoniazid	Methyldopa	Nabumetone
Norethandrolone	Oral contraceptives	Perphenazine
Phenazopyridine	Phenothiazine	Steroids
Sulfonamides	Tolmetin	

Medications that may cause false-negative results:
Ascorbic acid	Chlorhexidine	Indomethacin

Medications that may cause false-positive results:
Pyridium-like medications
Urochromes

Blood Urea Nitrogen (BUN)

Normal Values
Newborn:	3-12 mg/dL; 1.1–4.3 mmol/L (SI)
Infant/Child:	5-18 mg/dL; 1.8–6.4 mmol/L (SI)
Adults:	10-20 mg/dL; 3.6-7.1 mmol/L (SI)
Elderly:	slightly higher than for adults

Critical Values
> 100 mg/dL; 35.7 mmol/L (SI)

Nutritional Significance

BUN measures the amount of urea nitrogen in the blood. Urea is a by-product of protein metabolism. Ingested proteins are broken down in the liver into amino acids which are catabolized and free ammonia is formed. The ammonia is converted to urea and transported in the blood to the kidneys for excretion. The BUN level is directly related to the metabolic function of the liver and excretory function of the kidney. Individuals with an elevated BUN have azotemia. Slightly higher values of BUN seen in the elderly are often the result of dehydration or an inability to concentrate urine. If the BUN continues to increase it may indicate that the kidney function is declining. The BUN is interpreted in conjunction with the creatinine test to assess kidney excretory function. A BUN >100 mg/dL usually indicates serious kidney problems. Individuals with unilateral kidney disease may not have elevated BUN levels because the unaffected kidney compensates for the diseased kidney.

The BUN also increases in individuals on a high protein diet or who have gastrointestinal bleeding. Both result in excess

BLOOD UREA NITROGEN (BUN)

amounts of protein in the hepatic circulation and elevated BUN levels result. Dehydration also creates a temporary elevation of BUN and may be used as a measure of hydration status following surgery. Starvation is associated with elevated levels of BUN because visceral protein is broken down into amino acids at an accelerated rate, urea production increases and BUN accumulates.

Patients with an acute myocardial infarction will experience a rise in BUN because of the reduced cardiac function and diminished renal blood flow. Renal excretion of BUN is reduced and BUN levels rise. In patients with both kidney disease and liver disease (hepatorenal syndrome), the BUN may be elevated then return to normal. This does not suggest improved renal excretory function, but rather that the liver is unable to form urea. As the liver continues to decline, the blood ammonia levels will rise, while the BUN may remain normal or slightly elevated. In nephrotic syndrome there is protein loss in the urine. With protein depletion, BUN is reduced.

RELATED TESTS: creatinine, creatinine clearance, microalbumin

Increased with:
- **Pre-renal causes**
- Hypovolemia
- Anabolic steroid use
- Shock
- Congestive heart failure
- High protein intake
- Feeding tube

Decreased with:
- Impaired absorption
  - celiac disease
- Severe liver damage:
  - drugs
  - liver failure
  - poisoning
  - hepatitis

BLOOD UREA NITROGEN (BUN)

Increased with:
- Increased protein catabolism:
  - hemorrhage in GI
  - acute MI
  - stress
  - starvation
  - diabetes with DKA
  - fever
  - burns
- Impaired renal function
- **Renal causes:**
- urinary obstruction
- glomerulonephritis
- pyelonephritis
- acute tubular necrosis
- renal failure
- **Post Renal Causes:**
- ureteral obstruction
- bladder outlet obstruction

Decreased with:
- Increased protein synthesis
  - late pregnancy
  - infancy
  - acromegaly
- Negative Nitrogen balance:
  - low protein, high CHO diet
  - Malnutrition
- Nephrotic syndrome
- Overhydration due to:
  - fluid overload
  - SIADH syndrome

Medications that may increase levels:

ACE inhibitors	Acetaminophen	Acetazolamide
Acyclovir	Albendazole	Aldesleukin
Alkaline antacids	Allopurinol	Altretamine
Amantadine	Amikacin	Amiloride
Amino acids	Amiodarone	Amphotericin B
Amyl nitrite	Anabolic steroids	Aprepitant
Aripiprazole	Arsenicals	Asparaginase
Aspirin	Atenolol	Azathioprine
Azithromycin	Aztreonam	Bacitracin
Benazepril	Benzthiazide	Betaxolol
Bismuth subsalicylate	Bisoprolol	Busulfan

BLOOD UREA NITROGEN (BUN)

Medications that may increase levels:

Calcitriol	Candesartan	Cannabis
Capreomycin	Captopril	Carbamazepine
Carvedilol	Castro oil	Cefaclor
Cefamandole	Cefazolin	Cefixime
Cefonicid	Cefoperazone	Cefotaxime
Cefotetan	Cefoxitin	Cefpodoxime
Ceftazidime	Ceftibuten	Ceftizoxime
Ceftriaxone	Cefuroxime	Cephalexin
Cephalothin	Cetirizine	Chemotherapy
Chloroform	Chlorothiazide	Chlorpheniramine
Chlortetracycline	Chlorthalidone	Cimetidine
Cinoxacin	Ciprofloxacin	Cisplatin
Clarithromycin	Clindamycin	Clonidine
Clorazepate	Clotrimazole	Codeine
Colistin	Cotrimoxazole	Cyclosporine
Demeclocycline	Dexamethasone	Dextran
Diazepam	Diazoxide	Diclofenac
Disopyramide	Diuretics	Doxorubicin
Doxycycline	Enalapril	Eplerenone
Epoetin alfa	Eprosartan	Ergot preparations
Ethacrynic acid	Ethambutol	Ether
Ethosuximide	Etidronate	Etretinate
Fenoprofen	Flucytosine	Fludarabine
Flutamide	Foscarnet	Furosemide
Gabapentin	Ganciclovir	Gemcitabine
Gentamicin	Gold	Griseofulvin
Guanethidine	Hydralazine	Hydrochlorothiazide
Hydroflumethiazide	Hydroxyurea	Ibuprofen
Idarubicin	Ifosfamide	Imipramine
Immune globin	Indomethacin	Interleukin
Irbesartan	Iron	Isosorbide
Kanamycin	Ketoprofen	Ketorolac
Labetalol	Leuprolide	Levodopa
Levorphanol	Lisinopril	Lithium
Lomefloxacin	Loracarbef	Losartan
Meclofenamate	Mefenamic acid	Melphalan
Meropenem	Mesalamine	Methicillin
Methotrexate	Methsuximide	Methyclothiazide
Methyldopa	Methysergide	Metolazone
Metoprolol	Micardis	Minocycline
Misoprostol	Mitomycin	Mitoxantrone

Blood Urea Nitrogen (BUN)

Medications that may increase levels:

Moexipril	Molindone	Moxalactam
Nabumetone	Nalidixic acid	Naproxen
Neomycin	Netilmicin	Nifedipine
Nilutamide	Nisoldipine	Nitrofurantoin
Norfloxacin	Ofloxacin	Olsalazine
Oxacillin	Oxaprozin	Oxytetracycline
Pamidronate	Pargyline	Paromomycin
Paroxetine	Pegaspargase	Penicillamine
Penicillin	Pentamidine	Pentostatin
Phenazopyridine	Phosphorus	Piperacillin
Piroxicam	Plicamycin	Probenecid
Propafenone	Propranolol	Propylthiouracil
Quazepam	Quinapril	Quinethazone
Quinine	Radiographic agents	Ramipril
Rifampin	Risperidone	Ritonavir
Sargramostim	Semustine	Silver
Spectinomycin	Spironolactone	Streptokinase
Sulfamethoxazole	Sulfasalazine	Sulfisoxazole
Sulindac	Suprofen	Tacrolimus
Tetracycline	Thallium	Thiazides
Ticarcillin	Ticlopidine	Timolol
Tinzaparin	Tobramycin	Tolmetin
Trandolapril	Tretinoin	Triamterene
Trimethoprim	Trimetrexate	Trovafloxacin
Vancomycin	Vasopressin	Venlafaxine
Verapamil	Vitamin D	Zalcitabine
Zolpidem		

Medications that may decrease levels:

Amikacin	Ascorbic acid	Capreomycin
Cefotaxime	Chloramphenicol	Levodopa
Phenothiazine	Streptomycin	

C- Reactive Protein (CRP)
High Sensitivity- C-Reactive Protein

Normal Values: CRP
Adults: <1.0 mg/dL or < 10 mg/L (SI)

hs-CRP : Cardiac Risk
Low: < 1.0 mg/dL
Average: 1.0-3.0 mg/dL
High: > 3.0 mg/dL

Nutritional Significance of C-Reactive Protein

CRP is an acute-phase reactant protein produced by the liver under the control of interleukin-6. Serum levels increase in infectious diseases, inflammatory disorders, malignancy and tissue trauma. The synthesis of CRP is initiated by antigen-immune complexes, bacteria, fungi and trauma. It is functionally analogous to immunoglobin G, however it is not antigen specific. CRP is used to diagnose bacterial infectious disease and inflammatory disorders such as acute rheumatic fever and rheumatoid arthritis. However, levels do not consistently rise with viral infections. It is a more sensitive measure than erythrocyte sedimentation rate by demonstrating a more intense increase in the presence of acute inflammatory changes. As the patient recovers, CRP declines to normal more rapidly than erythrocyte sedimentation rate. It is also reduced when the inflammatory process is suppressed by salicylates or steroids. An increase in CRP is associated with decreased levels of albumin and prealbumin. A positive test indicates an acute inflammatory reaction but, it does not indicate the cause of the reaction.

This test is also used to monitor patients with a

C- REACTIVE PROTEIN (CRP)
HIGH SENSITIVITY- C-REACTIVE PROTEIN (hs- CRP)

myocardial infarction. The level of CRP follows a similar pattern to creatine kinase MB isoenzyme, however the peak occurs 1-3 days later. If CRP levels do not return to < 1.0 mg/dL, this suggests damage to heart tissue. Levels are not elevated with angina pectoris. CRP is used postoperatively to identify wound infections. Generally, CRP increases 4-6 hours after surgery and will return to <1.0 mg/dL in 3 days. Elevated levels suggest inflammation and possibly infection or pulmonary infarction.

NUTRITIONAL SIGNIFICANCE OF hs-C-REACTIVE PROTEIN

Several studies have shown that serum hs-CRP level maybe related to the risk of future CAD in healthy adults, even with normal lipids. Other studies have demonstrated that hs-CRP is a weak predictor of cardiovascular risk. Chronic inflammation develops in response to excessive damage to the endothelial lining of the arteries resulting in the proliferation of lipid filled macrophages, smooth muscle cells and cytokines. However, chronic inflammation may be from another source other than the vascular system. More research is needed to determine the value of hs-CRP as a predictor of CVD risk and future cardiovascular risk in patients with acute coronary syndromes. Some statin therapies have anti-inflammatory effects and are associated with lower levels of hs-CRP as well as improved lipid profiles.

Due to individual variation in hs-CRP values, 2 separate measurements are required to classify a person's risk level.

C- Reactive Protein (CRP)
High Sensitivity- C- Reactive Protein

Cigarette smoking can cause increased levels. Weight loss, moderate alcohol consumption and increased physical activity including endurance exercise can result in decreased levels.

Related Tests: ESR, fibrinogen, lipoproteins, homocysteine

Increased with:
- ↑ BMI
- ↓ HDL/ ↑TG
- Acute rheumatic fever
- Arthritis, rheumatoid
- Chronic Bacterial infection (gingivitis, bronchitis)
- Bacterial meningitis
- Cigarette smoking
- Crohn's disease
- Diabetes mellitus
- Hypertension
- Malignancy
- Metabolic syndrome
- Pulmonary infarction
- Reiter's syndrome
- Systemic lupus
- Tissue trauma
- Tuberculosis
- Urinary tract infection
- Vasculitis syndrome
- Wound infection

Decreased with:
- ↑ endurance exercise
- ↑ physical activity
- Moderate alcohol consumption
- Suppression of inflammatory response
- Weight loss

Medications that may increase levels:
oral contraceptives

Medications that may decrease levels:
Fibrates	NSAIDS	Statins
Niacin	Salicylates	Steroids

CALCIUM (Ca), BLOOD

NORMAL VALUES
TOTAL CALCIUM
< 10 days:	7.6-10.4 mg/dL; 1.9-2.6 mmol/L (SI)
10 days- 2 yr:	9. -10.6 mg/dL; 2.3-2.65 mmol/L (SI)
Child:	8.8-10.8 mg/dL; 2.2-2.7 mmol/L (SI)
Adult:	9.0-10.5 mg/dL; 2.25-2.6 mmol/L (SI)
Elderly:	values slightly decreased

IONIZED CALCIUM
Newborn:.	4.2 - 5.58 mg/dL; 1.05 - 1.39 mmol/L (SI)
2 mos- 18 yr:	4.8 - 5.52 mg/dL; 1.2 - 1.31 mmol/L (SI)
Adult:	4.5 - 5.6 mg/dL; 1.05 - 1.30 mmol/L (SI)
Elderly:	values slightly decreased

CRITICAL VALUES
TOTAL CALCIUM
< 6 mg/dL; <1.5 mmol/L OR > 13 mg/dL; > 3.2 mmol/L

IONIZED CALCIUM
< 2.2 mg/dL; <0.55 mmol/L OR > 7 mg/dL; > 1.75 mmol/L

NUTRITIONAL SIGNIFICANCE

The bone and teeth are the reservoir for approximately 99 percent of body calcium. Serum calcium is a vital component of numerous metabolic enzymatic pathways. It is necessary for muscle contractility, cardiac function, neural transmission and blood clotting. When blood levels decrease, parathyroid hormone (PTH) is released. Serum calcium level is used to evaluate parathyroid function and calcium metabolism. It is used to monitor individuals with renal failure, renal transplantation, hyperparathyroidism and some cancers. Critical values are <6 mg/dL; <1.5 mmol/L, possibly leading to tetany and >13 mg/dL; > 3.2 mmol/L possibly leading to cardiac arrest and coma.

Calcium (Ca), Blood

The total serum calcium value includes both ionized calcium and calcium bound to albumin. About 50 percent of all calcium exists in the blood as ionized calcium and 50 percent is bound to albumin. When the serum albumin is low, the serum calcium level will appear to be low. When the serum albumin is high the serum calcium level is elevated. The total serum calcium level decreases by about 0.8 mg for every 1 gm decrease in serum albumin. When serum albumin levels are low, the ionized form of calcium is measured. This test is not affected by changes in serum albumin. The ionized calcium test is considered to be a more reliable and sensitive measure of total calcium. It is used for the detection of primary hyperparathyroidism. However, not all laboratories have the equipment to perform the ionized calcium assay. Panic levels for ionized calcium are < 2.2 mg/dL; <0.5 mmol/L that may produce tetany and > 7.0 mg/dL; > 1.75 mmol/L that may cause coma.

The serum level of calcium must be elevated on three different blood draws for a diagnosis of hypercalcemia. The most common cause of hypercalcemia is hyperparathyroidism. Elevated calcium is due to the action of parathyroid hormone increasing gastrointestinal absorption, decreasing urinary excretion and increasing bone resorption.

Cancer is also a common cause of hypercalcemia. Tumor metastasis to the bone can promote bone resorption and raise serum calcium levels. There is a decreasing urinary excretion and

CALCIUM (Ca), BLOOD

increasing bone resorption in multiple myeloma, lung, breast and renal cell cancers. Other cancers can produce parathyroid hormone-like substances that cause an increase in serum calcium. Individuals who consume large amounts of vitamin D can have hypercalcemia due to increased renal and gastrointestinal absorption. Hypercalcemia is seen in tuberculosis and sarcoidosis.

Hypocalcemia is seen in conjunction with hypoalbuminemia due to malnutrition. Large-volume IV infusions may result in hypocalcemia because the citrate additives used in stored blood for anticoagulation bind the free calcium in the recipient's blood. Intestinal malabsorption, renal failure, rhabdomyolysis, alkalosis and acute pancreatitis are also associated with low serum calcium levels. Hypomagnesemia can be associated with refractory hypocalcemia.

Urinary calcium is one way to confirm a diagnosis of hypercalcemia. Excretion of calcium in the urine is increased in all patients with hypercalcemia. Excretion is reduced in patients with hypocalcemia.

RELATED TESTS: parathyroid hormone, albumin

Total Ca increased with:
- Hyperparathyroidism
- Metastatic tumor of bone
- Cancer of lung, breast, liver
- Cancer of thyroid, pancreas
- Hodgkin's disease
- Leukemia
- Non-Hodgkin's disease
- Multiple myeloma

Total Ca decreased with:
- Hypoparathyroidism
- Renal failure
- Pancreatitis
- Fat embolism
- Alkalosis
- Hepatic cirrhosis
- Vitamin D deficiency
- Rickets

CALCIUM (Ca), BLOOD

Total Ca increased with:
- Burkitt's lymphoma
- Primary squamous cell cancer of neck & head
- Thyroid toxicosis
- Excessive intake antacids
- Renal transplant
- Vitamin D intoxication
- Sarcoidosis
- Tuberculosis
- Milk-alkali syndrome
- Addison's disease
- Acromegaly
- Hyperthyroidism
- Paget's disease
- Prolonged immobilization

Total Ca decreased with:
- Osteomalacia
- Hyperphosphatemia secondary to renal failure
- Celiac disease
- Alcoholism
- Sprue
- Malabsorption
- Hypoalbuminemia

Ionized Ca increased with:
- Hyperparathyroidism
- Ectopic PTH-producing tumors
- Malignancies
- Increased vitamin D intake

Ionized Ca decreased with:
- Acute pancreatitis
- Administration of bicarbonate to control metabolic acidosis
- Hyperventilation to control increased intracranial pressure
- Hypoparathyroidism
- Vitamin D deficiency
- Magnesium deficiency
- Multiple organ failure
- Toxic shock syndrome

Medications that may increase levels:

Aldesleukin	Alkaline antacids	Aluminium
Anabolic steroids	Antacids	Basiliximab
Calcitriol	Calcium gluconate	Captopril
Cefotaxime	Chlorothiazide	Chlorpropamide
Chlorthalidone	Dienestrol	Diethylstilbestrol

CALCIUM (CA), BLOOD

Medications that may increase levels:

Dihydrotachysterol	Doxorubicin	Estramustine
Estropipate	Etretinate	Fluoxymesterone
Hydralazine	Hydrochlorothiazide	Iron
Leflunomide	Leuprolide	Levodopa
Lithium	Magnesium	Methyclothiazide
Methyltestosterone	Metoclopramide	Metolazone
Mycophenolate	Nandrolone	Nisoldipine
Oral contraceptives	Oxymetholone	Parathyroid hormone
Paroxetine	Pentostatin	Phenobarbital
Polystyrene sulfonate	Polythiazide	Progesterone
Propranolol	Riluzole	Sirolimus
Spironolactone	Tamoxifen	Theophylline
Thiazides	Toremifene	Trastuzumab
Tretinoin	Trichlormethiazide	Vitamin D
Zalcitabine		

Medications that may decrease levels:

Acetazolamide	Aldesleukin	Alendronate
Amifostine	Amlodipine	Amphotericin B
Anticonvulsants	Arsenic trioxide	Asparaginase
Aspirin	Basiliximab	Bisphosphonates
Calcitonin	Carbamazepine	Chloroquine
Chlorothiazide	Cidofovir	Cinacalcet
Cisplatin	Corticosteroids	Cortisone
Diuretics	Doxorubicin	Erythropoietin
Estrogen/progestin therapy	Estropipate	Etidronate
Etretinate	Famotidine	Felbamate
Foscarnet	Furosemide	Gallium
Gentamicin	Glucocorticoids	Hydrochlorothiazide
Insulin	Interferon	Iron dextran
Isoniazid	Ketoconazole	Laxatives
Magnesium salts	Methicillin	Mycophenolate
Oral contraceptives	Pamidronate	Paroxetine
Pentamidine	Phenobarbital	Phenytoin
Plicamycin	Polystyrene sulfonate	Prednisone
Probucol	Raloxifene	Sargramostim
Streptozocin	Tacrolimus	Tamoxifen
Tetracycline	Theophylline	Tobramycin
Trimetrexate	Zalcitabine	Zoledronic acid

CALCIUM (Ca), URINE

The calcium urine test is used to detect hypocalciuria or hypercalciuria. The test requires a 24 hour urine collection. Hypercalciuria, or excessive urinary calcium excretion, occurs in about 5-10 percent of the population. It is the most common identifiable cause of calcium kidney stone disease. There are several options to define hypercalciuria as noted on Tables 10-11. In some instances the dietary and supplemental calcium is restricted. Urine calcium values may be affected by the amount of calcium in the diet as noted in the Table 11 below.

TABLE 10. Definitions of Hypercalciuria

Nutrition Rx	Definitions
Unrestricted diet	Females:> 250 mg; 6.2 mmol calcium/ 24 hr
	Males: 275-300 mg; 7.5 mmol calcium/ 24 hr
	> 4 mg/kg body wt/24 hr OR
	200 mg of calcium per liter.
Restricted Diet: 400 mg Calcium, 100 mEq Na	> 3 mg/kg body wt/24 hr

TABLE 11. Expected Urine Calcium Ranges

Calcium in Diet	Expected Urine Calcium Ranges
Low	< 150 mg/24-hour sample or < 3.7 mmol/24 hr
Average	100-250 mg/24-hour sample or 2.5-6.2 mmol per day
High	250-300 mg/24-hour sample or 6.2-7.5 mmol

Absorptive hypercalciuria is the most common cause of excessive urinary calcium. About 50 percent of all calcium stone

Calcium (Ca), Urine

formers have some form of absorptive hypercalciuria related to an increase in the normal gastrointestinal absorption of calcium, overly aggressive vitamin D supplementation, or excessive ingestion of calcium-containing foods (milk-alkali syndrome). Calcium absorption occurs mainly in the duodenum and normally represents only about 20 percent of the dietary calcium intake.

There are several types of absorptive hypercalciuria. Type I is the most severe type and is relatively unresponsive to changes in dietary modifications, i.e. severe calcium restriction. Type II is the most common variety of absorptive hypercalciuria and usually responds to moderate dietary calcium restriction. Urinary calcium levels will normalize during fasting in both Types I and II.

Type III is also known as renal phosphate leak. The etiology of Type III is a renal defect that causes excessive urinary phosphate excretion resulting in hypophosphatemia. The low serum phosphate level increases the activation of vitamin D which increases absorption of both phosphate and calcium. The body excretes the unnecessary calcium. Phosphate leak is essentially an absorptive vitamin D-dependent hypercalciuria due to inappropriate vitamin D activation from hypophosphatemia. Renal leak hypercalciuria is due to a specific defect in the kidneys that allows excessive obligatory urinary calcium excretion regardless of serum calcium levels, body stores, or calcium ingestion. The calcium/creatinine ratio usually is high (>0.20). The obligatory loss of serum calcium into the urine produces a

CALCIUM (Ca), URINE

mild hypocalcemia and secondary hyperparathyroidism.

Resorptive hypercalciuria is due to the loss of calcium from the body's normal skeletal stores and typically is found in hyperparathyroidism. In this condition, calcium is released from bone in response to the increased activity of osteoclasts caused by excessive and inappropriate serum PTH levels resulting in significant hypercalcemia. Under normal conditions, PTH causes the kidney to limit calcium excretion. However, with the overwhelming serum calcium load produced with hyperparathyroidism, the kidneys excrete the extra calcium into the urine, causing the hypercalciuria. Increased calcium excretion is also associated with high sodium intakes. Each 100 mEq increase in daily sodium raises urinary calcium level by about 50 mg.

Low urine calcium levels may suggest kidney disease hypoparathyroidism, low dietary calcium and vitamin D, poor absorption of calcium or vitamin D or. Pregnant women and older men may also have low urine calcium levels.

RELATED TESTS: parathyroid hormone, serum calcium, serum phosphate, thyroid function tests, PTH

Increased with:
- Absorptive hypercalciuria
- Renal phosphate leak
- ↑ dietary calcium intake
- ↑ dietary vitamin D intake

- Thyrotoxicosis (hypertyhopridism)
- Hyperparathyroidism

Decreased with:
- Hypoparathyroidism
- ↓ dietary calcium intake
- ↓ dietary vitamin D intake
- Poor absorption of dietary calcium
- Poor absorption of dietary vitamin D
- Vitamin D deficiency

CALCIUM (Ca), URINE

Increased with:
- Addison disease
- Paget's disease
- Osteoporosis
- Dehydration
- Granulomatous diseases
- Excessive intake of calcium antacids
- Kidney disease
  - renal tubular acidosis
  - Albright tubular acidosis
- Glucocorticoid excess
- Paraneoplastic syndromes
- Prolonged immobilization
- Cancers
  - bone
  - leukemia
  - lymphoma
  - metastatic tumors
  - multiple myeloma
  - sarcoidosis
- Milk-alkali syndrome
- Hypervitaminosis A

Decreased with:
- Pregnancy
- Aging men
- Kidney disease
- Metabolic alkalosis
- Gitelman syndrome

Medications that may increase levels:

Acetazolamide	Aluminum hydroxide	Amiloride
Ammonium chloride	Antacids	Anticonvulsants
Ascorbic acid	Asparginase	Bumetanide
Calcitonin	Chlorothiazide	Cholestyramine
Clonazepam	Clorazepate	Corticosteroids
Corticotropin	Dexamethasone	Diazepam
Diltiazem	Dimercaprol	Diurteics
Doralamide	Ergocalciferol	Ethacrynic acid
Fenoldopam	Furosemide	Gluycocorticoids
Interferon	Lithium	Lorazepam
Mannitol	Methazolamide	Methyclothiazide

Calcium (Ca), Urine

Medications that may increase levels:

Metolazone	Nandrolone	Phenobarbital
Plicamycin	Prednisolone	Spironolactone
Topiramate	Torsemide	Triamcinolone
Triamterene	Vitamin D	Vitamin K

Medications that may decrease levels:

Adrenocorticosteroid	Alendronate	Bicarbonate
Bisphosphonates	Bortezomib	Calcitonin
Chloroquine'	Chlorothiazide	Cisplatin
Estrogen	Etidronate	Gallium nitrate
Hormone replacement therapy	Hydrochlorothiazide	Ibandronate
Ketoconazole	Lithium	Mestranol
Methyclothiazide	Neomycin	Octreotide
Oral contraceptives	Pamidronate	Parathyroid extract
Phenytoin	Polythiazide	Quinapril
Risedronate	Sodium oxybate	Spironolactone
Thiazides	Trichlormethiazide	Vitamin K
Zoledronic acid		

CHLORIDE

NORMAL VALUES

Premature infant:	95-110 mEq/L; 95-110 mmol/L (SI)
Newborn infant:	96-106 mEq/L; 96-106 mmol/L (SI)
Child:	90-110 mEq/L; 90-110 mmol/L (SI)
Adults/Elderly:	98-106 mEq/L; 98-106 mmol/L (SI)

NUTRITIONAL SIGNIFICANCE

Chloride is the major extracellular anion that works with sodium to maintain serum osmolality. Absorption of chloride depends on sodium reabsorption and is regulated by the secretion of aldosterone. Any changes in sodium reabsorption will secondarily impact the serum chloride level. In doing so, chloride affects acid-base balance, water balance and osmolality. Chloride's main purpose is to maintain electrical neutrality via the chloride shift. Chloride moves into and out of RBC in exchange for bicarbonate (HCO_3) to maintain acid-base balance. The carbonic acid formed in RBC separates into H and HCO_3. The hydrogen ion binds to hemoglobin leaving the HCO_3 free to move out of the RBC. The electrical neutrality is maintained by chloride shifting into the RBC.

Hypochloremia is almost always seen with hyponatremia. Signs and symptoms include hyperexcitability of the nervous system and muscles, shallow breathing, hypotension and tetany. As the chloride level drops, the HCO_3 reabsorption increases proportionately causing metabolic alkalosis. The abnormally high level of HCO_3 results in a shift of intercellular hydrogen out of the cell and potassium into the cell resulting in hypokalemia. Critical values are < 80 mEq/L.

CHLORIDE

Hyperchloremia is often seen with hypernatremia. Signs and symptoms include lethargy, weakness and deep breathing. As the chloride level increases, the HCO3 reabsorption decreases proportionately causing metabolic acidosis. Critical values are >115 mEq/L.

RELATED TESTS: sodium, potassium, HCO3, urine chloride

Increased with (hyperchloremia):
- Dehydration
- Renal tubular acidosis
- Cushing's syndrome
- Eclampsia
- Multiple myeloma
- Kidney dysfunction
- Metabolic acidosis
- Hyperventilation
- Anemia
- Hypernatremia
- Hyperparathyroidism
- Respiratory alkalosis
- Diabetes insipidus
- Salicylate intoxication

- Head injury with hypothalamic damage
- Excessive infusion of normal saline

Decreased with (hypochloremia):
- Overhydration
- Congestive heart disease
- SIADH
- Vomiting
- Chronic gastric suction
- Chronic diarrhea
- Chronic respiratory acidosis
- Salt-losing nephritis
- Addison's disease
- Burns
- Hyponatremia
- Metabolic alkalosis
- Diuretic therapy
- Hypokalemia
- Aldosteronism
- Acute intermittent porphyria
- High volume GI fistulae

Medications that may increase levels:

Acetazolamide	Acetylcysteine	Ammonium chloride
Amoxapine	Amphotericin B	Aspirin
Asparaginase	Cannabis	Carbamazepine
Carvedilol	Carmustine	Cefotaxime
Chloride salts	Chlorothiazide	Chlorpheniramine

CHLORIDE

Medications that may increase levels:
Cholestyramine	Corticosteroids	Cyclosporine
Diazoxide	Etretinate	Guanethidine
Hydrochlorothiazide	Hydrocortisone	Iodine
Ion exchange resins	Lithium	Methyclothiazide
Methyldopa	Methyltestosterone	Neostigmine
NSAIDS	Triamterene	

Medications that may decrease levels:
Aldosterone	Allopurinol	Amiloride
Ascorbic acid	Bicarbonate	Bumetanide
Cefotaxime	Chlorpropamide	Chlorthalidone
Corticosteroids	Corticotropin	Cortisone
Etretinate	Furosemide	Hydrochlorothiazide
Hydrocortisone	Hydroflumethiazide	Laxatives
Loop Diuretics	Mannitol	Methyclothiazide
Metolazone	Polythiazide	Prednisone
Thiazides	Triamterene	Trimethoprim

CHOLESTEROL, TOTAL SERUM, LDL, HDL & VLDL

NORMAL FASTING VALUES: TOTAL CHOLESTEROL
Newborn: 53-135 mg/dL; 1.37-3.5 mmol/L (SI)
Infant: 70-175 mg/dL; 1.8-4.5 mmol/L (SI)

Children & Adolescents (12-18 yrs)
Desirable level: <170 mg/dL; < 4.4 mmol/L (SI)
Borderline High: 170-199 mg/dL; 4.4-5.2 mmol/L (SI)
High: > 240 mg/dL; > 6.2 mmol/L (SI)

Adult:
Desirable level: 140-199 mg/dL; 3.6-5.15 mmol/L (SI)
Borderline High: 200-239 mg/dL; 5.2-6.2 mmol/L (SI)
High: > 240 mg/dL; > 6.2 mmol/L (SI)

NORMAL FASTING VALUES: LDL
Children & Adolescents (12-18 yrs)
Desirable level: <110 mg/dL; < 2.8 mmol/L (SI)
Borderline High: 110-129 mg/dL; 2.8-3.4 mmol/L (SI)
High: > 130 mg/dL; > 3.4 mmol/L (SI)

Adult:
Desirable level: < 130 mg/dL; < 3.4 mmol/L (SI)
Borderline High: 140-159 mg/dL; 3.4-4.1 mmol/L (SI)
High: > 160 mg/dL; > 4.1 mmol/L (SI)

NORMAL FASTING VALUES: HDL
Adult Males: 35-65 mg/dL; 0.9-1.7 mmol/L (SI)
Adult Females: 35-80 mg/dL: 0.9-2.1 mmol/L (SI)

Normal values vary by age, diet, gender and geographical or cultural region.

NUTRITIONAL SIGNIFICANCE: TOTAL CHOLESTEROL

  Coronary artery disease (CAD) is a leading cause of morbidity and mortality in the United States and other developed

CHOLESTEROL, TOTAL SERUM, LDL, HDL & VLDL

countries. Attempts to determine the risk of heart attack and stroke based on a single criterion such as total cholesterol levels in different population groups have had limited success. For example, a follow-up to the Framingham study found that nearly half of the cases of CAD occurred in people with normal serum cholesterol. An abnormal lipid profile remains one of the most discriminating factors for the early detection of CAD.

Cholesterol is the main lipid associated with CAD. The plasma cholesterol level is a reflection of dietary intake and absorption, endogenous synthesis and excretion. Endogenous cholesterol is synthesized primarily in the liver and intestines. An adult male produces approximately 1 gm of cholesterol per day. Cholesterol can also be synthesized from acetyl coenzyme A in many tissues in the body. It is required for the production of steroids, bile acids and cellular membranes. The liver metabolizes cholesterol to its free form and lipoproteins transport cholesterol in the bloodstream. Approximately 75 percent of all cholesterol is bound to LDL and about 25 percent is bound to HDL. LDL level is most directly associated with increased risk of CAD.

Using electrophoresis, the lipoproteins are categorized as chylomicrons (primarily triglycerides), LDLs (primarily cholesterol), VLDLs (primarily triglycerides) and HDLs (primarily protein). The most accurate results for total serum cholesterol and lipoprotein levels are following a 12-14 hour fast. Based on the test results, many adults have restricted their dietary intake of fat and

Cholesterol, Total Serum, LDL, HDL & VLDL

cholesterol in hopes of reducing their risk of CAD. Strategies to lower serum cholesterol include dietary restriction of saturated fats and cholesterol, increased intake of insoluble fiber, exercise, weight loss and pharmacological intervention to increase fecal excretion of cholesterol. Current research suggests that CAD is a multifactorial condition.

LDL & VLDL

The majority of cholesterol (around 75 percent) is bound to LDL. The role of LDL is to carry cholesterol for deposit in peripheral tissues. Degradation of VLDL is the primary source of LDL. LDL levels are determined using this formula:

$$LDL = Total\ cholesterol - (HDL + TG/5)$$

This formula is only valid if the cholesterol and triglycerides are from a fasting specimen and the triglyceride level is less than 400 mg/dL; 4.5 mmol/L.

High levels of free and bound LDL are associated with an increased risk for CAD. LDL has a longer half-life (3-4 days) than its precursor VLDL, so it is more prevalent in the blood. LDL subfraction testing has been studied to determine if the number and type of LDL particles (LDL-P) predict the risk for CAD. Currently there is no reference method for evaluating LDL subfractions or standardization among the different methods used to measure LDL subfractions. A systematic review of the relationship between LDL subfractions and clinical cardiovascular outcomes concluded that the increased number of LDL-P and

CHOLESTEROL, TOTAL SERUM, LDL, HDL & VLDL

selected LDL subfractions may be associated with the incidence and progression of heart disease, but it is unclear whether the associations are dependent of current risk factors. Randomized trails are needed to validate the added value of these measures.

VLDL is synthesized in the liver and they transport endogenously synthesized triglycerides to adipose tissue for storage. The VLDL is usually expressed as a percentage of total cholesterol. Levels in excess of 25 to 50 percent are associated with increased risk of CAD.

HDL

Approximately 25 percent of the cholesterol is bound to HDL. The role of HDL is to transport cholesterol from peripheral tissues to the liver for excretion. HDLs may have a protective effect by preventing uptake of cholesterol and lipids at the cellular level. The HDL to total cholesterol ratio should be at least 1:5. High levels of HDL are associated with a decreased risk of coronary heart disease. The ideal HDL to cholesterol ratio is 1:3.

TABLE 12. HDL Levels & Risk for Coronary Artery Disease

HDL Ranges	Associated Risk
< 25 mg/dL; < 0.65 mmol/L	dangerous level, 2 X risk
26-35 mg/dL; 0.67-0.91 mmol/L	high risk, 1.5 X risk
36-44 mg/dL; 0.93-1.14 mmol/L	moderate risk, 1.2 X risk
45-59 mg/dL; 1.16-1.53 mmol/L	average risk
60-74 mg/dL; 1.55-1.92 mmol/L	below average risk
> 75 mg/dL; 1.94 mmol/L	no risk, associated with longevity

RELATED TESTS: Apo A-I, Apo B, hs-CRP, triglycerides

CHOLESTEROL, TOTAL SERUM, LDL, HDL & VLDL

Cholesterol Increased with:	Cholesterol Decreased with:

■ Coronary Artery Disease
  • hypercholesterolemia
  • hyperlipidemia
  • atherosclerosis
  • hypertension
■ Obesity
■ High cholesterol/fat diet
■ Xanthomatosis
■ Werner's syndrome
■ Hypothyroidism
■ Uncontrolled DM
■ Pregnancy
■ Stress
■ Cholestasis
■ Biliary cirrhosis
■ Alcoholism
■ Pancreatic & prostatic cancer
■ CRF
■ Nephrotic syndrome
■ Nephrosis
■ Glomerulonephritis
■ Glycogen storage disease
	■ Malabsorption
	■ Malnutrition
	■ Hypo-α–lipoproteinemia
	■ Advanced cancers
	■ Hyperthyroidism
	■ Burns
	■ Inflammation
	■ Sepsis
	■ Stress
	■ Liver disease
	■ AIDS
	■ Acute illness/infection
	■ Anemias
	  • pernicious anemia
	  • hemolytic anemia
	  • sideroblastic
	■ Myeloproliferative diseases
	■ COPD
	■ Acute MI
	■ Mental retardation

Medications that may increase serum cholesterol levels:

Acetohexamide	Acetophenazine	ACTH
Adalimumab	Alitretinoin	Aminoglutethimide
Amiodarone	Amphotericin B	Amprenavir
Anabolic steroids	Anastrazole	Antibiotics
Antihypertensives	Asparaginase	Aspirin
Atazanavir	Atenolol	Azathioprine
Basiliximab	Beclomethasone	Beta blockers
Betaxolol	Bicalutamide	Bisoprolol
Calcitriol	Captopril	Carbamazepine
Carvedilol	Cefotaxime	Chenodiol
Chlorothiazide	Chlorpromazine	Chlorpropamide
Chlorthalidone	Clofibrate	Clonidine
Clopidogrel	Conjugated estrogens	

Cholesterol, Total Serum, LDL, HDL & VLDL

Medications that may increase serum cholesterol levels:

Corticosteroids	Cortisone	Cyclophosphamide
Cyclosporine	Danazol	Dantrolene
Dapsone	Dextran	Diazepam
Diclofenac	Disulfiram	Efavirenz
Enalapril	Epinephrine	Eplerenone
Escitalopram	Ethanol	Ether
Etretinate	Fluoxymesterone	Fluvoxamine
Fosinopril	Furosemide	Gabapentin
Glyburide	Gold	Heparin
Hydrochlorothiazide	Ibandronate	Ibuprofen
Imipramine	Indapamide	Isotretinoin
Lansoprazole	Levarterenol	Lisinopril
Lithium	Medroxyprogesterone	Mepazine
Meprobamate	Methimazole	Methyclothiazide
Methyltestosterone	Miconazole	Mirtazapine
Mycophenolate	Nafarelin	Nandrolone
Naproxen	Nefazodone	Norethandrolone
Norfloxacin	Norplant	Ofloxacin
Olmesartan	Oral contraceptives	Oxymetholone
Paroxetine	Penicillamine	Pergolide
Phenobarbital	Phenothiazine	Phenytoin
Pindolol	Polythiazide	Pravastatin
Prednisolone	Prochlorperazine	Promazine
Propranolol	Radioactive iodine	Riluzole
Ritonavir	Rosiglitazone	Sargramostim
Sirolimus	Sodium oxybate	Sotalol
Spironolactone	Sulfadiazine	Sulfonamides
Tamoxifen	Testosterone	Tetracycline
Theophylline	Thiabendazole	Thiazides
Thiouracil	Ticlopidine	Tolcapone
Tretinoin	Trifluoperazine	Troglitazone
Venlafaxine	Vitamin A	Vitamin C
Vitamin D	Vitamin E	Zolpidem

Medications that may decrease serum cholesterol levels:

Acarbose	Acebutolol	Albuterol
Aldesleukin	Allopurinol	Aluminum hydroxide
Amikacin	Amiloride	Aminosalicylic acid
Amiodarone	Amlodipine	Ampicillin
Ascorbic acid	Asparaginase	Aspirin
Atenolol	Atorvastatin	Azathioprine

CHOLESTEROL, TOTAL SERUM, LDL, HDL & VLDL

Medications that may decrease serum cholesterol levels:

Bisoprolol	Captopril	Carvedilol
Chlorambucil	Chloroform	Chlorpropamide
Chlorthalidone	Cholestyramine	Cilazapril
Clofibrate	Clomiphene	Clonidine
Coenzyme Q10	Colchicine	Colestipol
Conjugated estrogens	Diltiazem	Dobutamine
Doxazocin	Doxazosin	Enalapril
Erythromycin	Esterified estrogens	Fenofibrate
Fluoxymesterone	Fluvastatin	Fosinopril
Gemfibrozil	Glyburide	Green tea
Granulocyte colonizing factor	HMG CoA-reductase inhibitors	Guanabenz
Haloperidol	Heparin (LMP, LMW)	Hydralazine
Hydroxychloroquine	Indomethacin	Insulin
Isoniazid	Isosorbide dinitrate	Isosorbide mononitrate
Isotretinoin	Isradipine	Kanamycin
Ketoconazole	Lansoprazole	Levonorgestrel
Levothyroxine	Lincomycin	Lisinopril
Losartan	MAO inhibitors	Medroxyprogesterone
Metformin	Methyldopa	Metoprolol
Metronidazole	Nandrolone	Neomycin
Niacin	Nicotinic acid	Nifedipine
Nitroglycerin	Norplant	Oral contraceptives
Orlistat	Oxandrolone	Oxymetholone
Pentamidine	Perindopril	Phenytoin
Pindolol	Pravastatin	Prazosin
Prednisolone	Probucol	Progesterone
Psyllium	Raloxifene	Ramipril
Simvastatin	Spironolactone	Statins
Streptokinase	Tacrolimus	Tamoxifen
Terazosin	Tetracycline	Thiazides
Thyroid	Tolbutamide	Tolcapone
Trazodone	Ursodiol	Valproic acid
Verapamil		

HDL Increased with:
- Long term aerobic and vigorous exercise

HDL Decreased with:
- Metabolic syndrome
- Familial low HDL

CHOLESTEROL, TOTAL SERUM, LDL, HDL & VLDL

HDL Increased with:
- Familial HDL lipoproteinemia
- Chronic liver disease
  - cirrhosis
  - alcoholism
  - hepatitis

HDL Decreased with:
- Poorly controlled DM
- Hypertriglyceridemia
- Hepatocellular disease
- Malnutrition
- Uremia
- CRF
- Nephrotic syndrome
- Cholestasis
- Smoking

LDL & VLDL Increased with:
- Familial hypercholesterolemia
- Chronic liver disease
- Glycogen storage disease
- Hypothyroidism
- High fat diet
- Obesity
- Poorly controlled DM
- Porphyria
- High alcohol consumption
- CRF
- Nephrotic syndrome
- Glomerulonephritis
- Multiple myeloma
- Pancreatic & prostatic cancers
- Hepatoma
- Cholestasis
- Alcoholism
- Biliary cirrhosis

LDL & VLDL Decreased with:
- Familial hypolipoproteinemia
- Malnutrition
- Malabsorption
- Hyperthyroidism
- Apo C-II deficiency
- Chronic anemias
- Severe hepatocellular disease
- Burns
- Inflammatory joint disease
- Reye's syndrome
- Myeloproliferative diseases
- Acute illness, infection
- COPD

Medications that may increase lipoproteins

Alpha-blockers	Beta-blockers	Dilantin
Estrogen	Aspirin	Oral contraceptives
Phenothiazine	Steroids	Sulfonamides

CORTISOL, BLOOD & URINE

NORMAL BLOOD VALUES
Newborn:	1-24 mcg/dL; 28-662 nmol/L (SI)
Child 1-16 yr 8 AM:	3–21 mcg/dL; 83-579 nmol/L (SI)
Child 1-16 yr 4 PM:	3–10 mcg/dL; 83-276 nmol/L (SI)
Adult/Elderly 8 AM:	5–23 mcg/dL; 138-635 nmol/L (SI)
Adult/Elderly 4 PM:	3–13 mcg/dL; 83-359 nmol/L (SI)

NORMAL URINE VALUES (24 HR SPECIMEN)
Child:	2-27 mcg/24 hr; 5.52-74.5 nmol/24 hr (SI)
Adolescent:	5-55 mcg/24 hr; 13.8-151.7 nmol/24 hr (SI)
Adult/Elderly:	< 100 mcg/24 hr; 276 nmol/24 hr (SI)

NUTRITIONAL SIGNIFICANCE

Cortisol is a glucocorticosteroid synthesized in the cortex of the adrenal glands from cholesterol. Levels of cortisol affect the metabolism of protein, carbohydrate and fat. Cortisol stimulates gluconeogenesis by the liver and inhibits the effect of insulin thereby decreasing the rate of glucose use by cells. In healthy adults, the secretion of cortisol is higher early in the morning (6:00-8:00 AM) and lower in the evening (4:00-6:00 PM). Normal values may be transposed in individuals who have worked during the night and slept during the day for long periods. This diurnal variation is lost in patients with Cushing's syndrome and in persons under physical or emotional stress. Increasing levels of the cytokine TFN -α cause cortisol excess by releasing corticotrophin-releasing hormone which leads to muscle wasting.

In individuals with Cushing's syndrome as well as those with some types of cancer, cortisol levels are very high in the morning, but there is no variation later in the day. Malignant

Cortisol, Blood & Urine

tumors may trigger the overproduction of ACTH. The best method of evaluating adrenal activity is by directly measuring plasma cortisol levels. However, urine cortisol levels may be used if 24 hour urine specimen is available.

Related Tests: ACTH, cortisol suppression, glucose

Increased with:
- Hyperthyroidism
- Trauma
- Surgery
- Carcinoma
- Cushing's syndrome
- Physical or emotional stress
- Overproduction of ACTH
- Adrenal adenoma
- Obesity

Decreased with:
- Adrenal hyperplasia
- Addison's disease
- Hypopituitarism
- Hypothyroidism
- Liver disease
- Anterior pituitary hyposecretion

Medications that may increase plasma cortisol:

Amphetamines	Anticonvulsants	Aspirin
Atropine	Benzodiazepines	Citalopram
Clomipramine	Corticotropin	Corticotropin-releasing hormone
Cortisone	Diazoxide	Diclofenac
Estrogen	Ether	Ethinyl estradiol
Fenoprofen	Furosemide	Gemfibrozil
Glyburide	Hydrocortisone	Insulin
Interferon	Interleukin	Lithium
Methadone	Methoxamine	Metoclopramide
Naloxone	Octreotide	Opiates
Oral contraceptives	Prednisolone	Prednisone
Ranitidine	Spironolactone	Tumor necrosis factor
Vasopressin		

CORTISOL, BLOOD & URINE

Medications that may decrease plasma cortisol:

Aminoglutethimide	Androgens	Barbiturates
Beclomethasone	Betamethasone	Budesonide
Clonidine	Corticosteroids	Danazol
Dexamethasone	Dextroamphetamine	Diazoxide
Ephedrine	Etomidate	Fluocinolone
Indomethacin	Ketoconazole	Labetalol
Levodopa	Lithium	Magnesium sulfate
Medroxyprogesterone	Megestrol	Mesalamine
Methylprednisolone	Metyrapone	Midazolam
Morphine	Nifedipine	Nitrous oxide
Norethindrone	Oxazepam	Phenobarbital
Phenytoin	Pravastatin	Prednisolone
Prednisone	Ranitidine	Rifampin
Steroids	Sumatriptan	Triamcinolone
Trimipramine		

CREATINE KINASE (CK) (formerly Creatine Phosphokinase CPK)

NORMAL VALUES
TOTAL CK
Newborns: 68-580 U/L; 68-580 U/L(SI)
Adult/Elderly: Male: 55-170 U/L; 55 - 170 U/L(SI)
Female: 30-135 U/L; 30 - 135 U/L(SI)

ISOENZYMES
CK-MM - 100%
CK-MB - 0%
CK-BB - 0%

NUTRITIONAL SIGNIFICANCE

CK is an enzyme found in the heart muscle, skeletal muscle and brain. Elevations in serum CK are always due to damaged muscle cells. The CK levels rise within 6 hours after trauma, peak at 18 hours and return to normal in 2 to 3 days if no additional injury occurs. Elevations in CK are often associated with a myocardial infarction, but the more sensitive troponins are used for diagnosis. To test specifically for a myocardial muscle injury three isoenzymes (CK-MM or CK3, CK-MB or CK2 and CK-BB or CK1) are evaluated. The CK-MB appears to be specific for myocardial cells. The CK-BB isoenzyme is primarily found in the brain and lung. Elevations in the CK-BB are associated with a cerebrovascular accident or pulmonary infarction.

The CK-MM isoenzyme normally makes up almost all of the circulatory total CK enzymes in healthy adults. When the CK level increases due to an elevation in CK-MM, it is likely due to disease, injury or stress to the skeletal muscle. Examples of this include myopathies, vigorous exercise, multiple MI injections,

CREATINE KINASE (CK) (formerly Creatine Phosphokinase CPK)

trauma, electroconvulsive therapy, cardioversion, chronic alcoholism and surgery. The normal value for CK-MM will be higher in larger muscular individuals.

Related Tests: AST, LDH, ALT, LAP, GGTP, ALP, 5' nucleotidase, troponin

CK Increased with:
- Acute MI
- Acute cerebrovascular disease
- Electric shock
- Convulsions
- Muscular dystrophy
- Dermatomyositis
- Chronic alcoholism
- Delirium tremens
- Polymyositis
- Hypokalemia
- CNS trauma
- Pulmonary infarction
- Malignant hyperthermia
- Reye's syndrome
- Hypothyroidism
- Neoplasm of prostate, bladder or GI tract
- Myocarditis
- Rhabdomyolysis with cocaine intoxication
- Acute psychosis
- Open heart surgery
- Eosinophilia-myalgia syndrome

CK -BB Increased with:
- Pulmonary infarction
- Electroconvulsive therapy
- Cerebrovascular accident
- Shock
- Adenocarcinoma
- Intestinal ischemia
- Pulmonary embolism
- Brain injury
- Seizures
- Reye's syndrome
- Muscle trauma
- Severe shock syndrome
- Neurosurgery
- Hypothermia
- Subarachnoid hemorrhage
- Neoplasm of breast, lung, bladder, uterus, testis, prostate

CK-MB Increased with:
- Acute MI
- Cardiac aneurysm
- Cardiac ischemia

CK -MM Increased with:
- Electroconvulsive therapy
- Myositis
- Delirium tremens

CREATINE KINASE (CK) (formerly Creatine Phosphokinase CPK)

CK-MB Increased with:
- Cardiac defibrillation
- Myocarditis
- Ventricular arrhythmias
- Reye's syndrome
- Muscular dystrophy
- Subarachnoid hemorrhage
- Muscle trauma, surgery
- Chronic renal failure
- Malignant hyperthermia
- Malignant hypothermia
- CO poisoning
- Polymyositis
- Myoglobulinemia
- Rocky Mountain spotted fever

CK -MM Increased with:
- Muscular dystrophy
- Recent convulsions
- Electromyography
- Hypokalemia
- Recent surgery
- Hypothyroidism
- Shock
- IM injections
- Crushing injuries, trauma
- Hemophilia
- Malignant hyperthermia
- Rhabdomyolysis

Medications that may increase levels:

5-Fluorouracil	Albuterol	Alcohol
Aminocaproic acid	Amoxapine	Amphotericin B
Ampicillin (IM)	Analgesics (IM)	Aripiprazole
Aspirin	Atorvastatin	Azithromycin
Candesartan	Captopril	Carbenicillin
Carteolol	Cefotaxime	Ceftizoxime
Cerivastatin	Chlordane	Chlordiazepoxide
Chloroform	Chlorothiazide	Chlorpromazine
Chlorthalidone	Cholestyramine	Clindamycin
Clofibrate	Clonidine	Clozapine
Colchicine	Cyclosporin	Danazol
Dantrolene	Dapsone	Dexamethasone
Diclofenac	Didanosine	Digoxin
Diltiazem	Diuretics (IM)	Donepezil
Ethchlorvynol	Etidocaine	Etretinate
Fenofibrate	Fluvastatin	Foscarnet
Furosemide	Ganciclovir	Gemfibrozil
Haloperidol	Hydrocortisone	Insulin
Interleukin	Isotretinoin	Itraconazole
Labetalol	Lamivudine	Levamisole
Lidocaine	Lithium	Lovastatin

CREATINE KINASE (CK) (formerly Creatine Phosphokinase CPK)

Medications that may increase levels:

Loxapine	Meperidine	Morphine (IM)
Narcotics (IM)	Nelfinavir	Niacin
Nifedipine	Nisoldipine	Olanzapine
Oral contraceptives	Paroxetine	Penicillamine
Penicillin	Phenelzine	Phenothiazine
Phenytoin	Pindolol	Pioglitazone
Pramipexole	Pravastatin	Prazosin
Probucol	Procainamide	Promethazine
Propranolol	Quinidine	Risperidone
Ritonavir	Simvastatin	Sirolimus
Tolcapone	Trimethoprim	Troglitazone
Tubocurarine	Vasopressin	Zalcitabine
Zidovudine		

Medications that may decrease levels:

Acetylsalicylic acid	Amikacin	Ascorbic acid
Calcium	Dantrolene	Dexamethasone
Droperidol	Phenothiazine	Pindolol
Prednisone	Sulfamethoxazole	

CREATININE CLEARANCE

NORMAL VALUES
Newborn: 40-65 mL/min; 0.67 – 1.1 mL/s (SI)
Adults: Male, < 40 yr: 107 - 139 mL/min; 1.78 – 2.32 mL/s (SI)
Female, < 40 yr: 87 - 107 mL/min; 1.45-1.78 mL/s (SI)

NUTRITIONAL SIGNIFICANCE

The creatinine clearance test is used to evaluate glomerular filtration rate (GFR) in terms of milliliters of filtrate produced by the kidneys per minute or per second. Creatinine is entirely excreted by the kidneys. It is directly proportional to the GFR. The creatinine clearance test is used to assess the ability of the glomeruli to act as a filter. Creatinine clearance is calculated using the number of milligrams per deciliter of creatinine excreted in 24 hours, the volume of urine in 24 hours and the serum creatinine. It requires a 24 hour urine collection and a serum creatinine level. The National Kidney Disease Education Program (NKDEP) recommends that clinical laboratories report an estimated GFR when reporting serum creatinine. Refer to Table 13.

$$\text{Creatinine Clearance} = \frac{UV}{P}$$

U = number of mg/dL creatinine excreted in urine over 24 hrs
V = volume of urine in mL/min
P = serum creatinine in mg/dL

Conditions which impact the results include a decrease in blood present for filtration and an inability of the glomeruli to act as a filter. A decrease in blood present for filtration can be due to renal artery atherosclerosis, dehydration or shock. Diseases

CREATININE CLEARANCE

affecting the glomeruli include glomerulonephritis, acute tubular necrosis and other primary renal diseases.

TABLE 13. Mean Estimated GFR Rates

Age (yrs)	Mean eGFR
20-29	116 mL/min/1.73 m^2
30-29	107 mL/min/1.73 m^2
40-49	99 mL/min/1.73 m^2
50-59	93 mL/min/1.73 m^2
60-69	85 mL/min/1.73 m^2
70+	75 mL/min/1.73 m^2

Individuals with unilateral kidney disease may not have a decrease in creatinine clearance levels because the unaffected kidney compensates for the diseased kidney. Creatinine clearance is affected by several non-renal factors. The rate decreases about 6.5 mL/min for each decade of age after age 20 years. Also muscle mass typically decreases with age giving lower creatinine clearance values. Individuals consuming large quantities of protein or creatine supplements may temporarily increase creatinine clearance values. Exercise may also increase values. Incomplete urine collection may give falsely low values.

RELATED TESTS: BUN, creatinine

Increased with:
- Exercise
- High cardiac output syndromes
- Pregnancy

Decreased with:
- Congestive heart failure
- COPD
- Cirrhosis with ascites
- Shock

CREATININE CLEARANCE

Increased with:
- CO poisoning
- Burns

Decreased with:
- Hemorrhage
- Dehydration
- Renal disease/injury
  - nephrotic syndrome
  - chronic nephritis
  - obstruction of urinary tract
  - acute tubular necrosis
  - glomerulonephritis
  - reduced renal blood flow
  - pyelonephritis
  - amyloidosis
  - interstitial nephritis

Medications that may increase levels:

Aminoglycosides	Ascorbic acid	Cefoxitin
Cephalosporins	Cephalothin	Cimetidine
Cisplatin	Corticosteroids	Fluoxymestrone
Gentamicin	Methotrexate	Methyldopa
Nandrolone	Nitrofurantoin	Nitrofurazone
Oxymetholone	Prednisone	

Medications that may decrease levels:

Anabolic steroids	Captopril	Cephalosporins
Cimetidine	Ketoprofen	Nandrolone
Prednisone	Quinapril	Thiazides
Trimethoprim		

CREATININE, SERUM

NORMAL VALUES
Newborn: 0.3-1.2 mg/dL; 27-106 μmol/L (SI)
Child: 0.3–0.7 mg/dL; 27-62 μmol/L (SI)
Adolescent: 0.5-1.0 mg/dL; 44-88 μmol/L (SI)
Adult males: 0.6-1.2 mg/dL; 53-106 μmol/L (SI)
Adult females: 0.5-1.1 mg/dL; 44-97 μmol/L (SI)
Elderly: slightly decreased with muscle atrophy

NUTRITIONAL SIGNIFICANCE

Creatinine is a by-product of the metabolism of muscle creatine phosphate to form ATP. It is produced at a constant rate determined by the individual's muscle mass and excretory function of the kidney. Often creatinine levels are slightly lower in the elderly due to decreased muscle mass.

An elevated creatinine suggests rapid muscle loss from trauma or surgery. Injury to skeletal muscles causes myoglobin to be released in the blood. Creatinine levels are increased in diseases associated with increased muscle mass such as acromegaly or gigantism. Elevated levels also indicate possible renal disorders. Slight increases may be seen after ingestion of large quantities of meat. Creatine supplementation to increase muscular strength/power may have adverse effects on creatinine if renal status is marginal or poor. Critical values > 4 mg/dL indicate serious impairment in renal function. However, a normal creatinine does not always mean unimpaired renal function. For example, in elderly or sedentary individuals the creatinine may be below normal ranges or normal due to muscle wasting. Creatinine levels are below normal ranges in diseases associated with

CREATININE, SERUM

decreased muscle mass such as muscular dystropy. Creatinine level is interpreted in conjunction with BUN. Unlike the BUN, creatinine is not significantly affected by dehydration, malnutrition or hepatic function.

RELATED TESTS: BUN, creatinine clearance

Increased with:
- Rapid muscle loss
- Surgery
- Trauma
- Diabetic nephropathy
- Rhabdomyolysis
- Renal disease/injury
  - azotemia
  - chronic nephritis
  - obstruction of urinary tract
  - acute tubular necrosis
  - glomerulonephritis
  - pyelonephritis
- Hyperthyroidism
- Atherosclerosis
- Shock
- Dehydration
- Congestive heart disease
- Acromegaly
- Gigantism

Decreased with:
- Muscular dystrophy
- Debilitation
- Decreased muscle mass
- Advanced liver disease
- Poliomyelitis
- Inadequate dietary protein

Medications that may increase levels:

ACE inhibitors	Acebutolol	Acetaminophen
Acetohexamide	Acyclovir	Adefovir
Albendazole	Aldesleukin	Alkaline antacids
Alprazolam	Alprostadil	Altretamine
Amikacin	Amiloride	Amiodarone
Ammonium chloride	Amoxapine	Amphotericin B
Aprepitant	Ascorbic acid	Asparaginase

CREATININE, SERUM

Medications that may increase levels:

Aspirin	Atenolol	Azathioprine
Azithromycin	Aztreonam	Barbiturates
Benazepril	Benzthiazide	Betaxolol
Bicalutamide	Bisoprolol	Candesartan
Capreomycin	Captopril	Carbamazepine
Carvedilol	Caspofungin	Cefaclor
Cefadroxil	Cefamandole	Cefazolin
Cefepime	Cefixime	Cefoperazone
Cefotaxime	Cefotetan	Cefoxitin
Cefpodoxime	Cefprozil	Ceftazidime
Ceftibuten	Ceftizoxime	Ceftriaxone
Cefuroxime	Cephalexin	Cephaloridine
Cephalothin	Cephradine	Cetirizine
Chlorothiazide	Chlorpropamide	Chlorthalidone
Cidofovir	Cimetidine	Cinoxacin
Ciprofloxacin	Cisplatin	Clarithromycin
Clindamycin	Clofibrate	Clonidine
Clorazepate	Clofarabine	Codeine
Colistimethate	Colistin	Cotrimoxazole
Cyclosporine	Danazol	Demeclocycline
Dexrazoxane	Dextran	Diclofenac
Didanosine	Disopyramide	Diuretics
Dopamine	Doxorubicin	Doxycycline
Enalapril	Enflurane	Eplerenone
Epoetin alfa	Eprosartan	Ethambutol
Etidronate	Etretinate	Fenoprofen
Flucytosine	Fludarabine	Fluoxymesterone
Foscarnet	Furosemide	Gabapentin
Ganciclovir	GCSF	Gemcitabine
Gemfibrozil	Gentamicin	Glycerin
Griseofulvin	Hetastarch	Hydralazine
Hydrochlorothiazide	Hydroxychloroquine	Hydroxyurea
Ibuprofen	Idarubicin	Imatinib
Imipramine	Immune globin	Indomethacin
Interleukin	Interleukin alfa-2	Irbesartan
Isotretinoin	Kanamycin	Ketoprofen
Ketorolac	Labetalol	Lactulose
Lamotrigine	Lansoprazole	Leuprolide
Levodopa	Lidocaine	Lisinopril
Lithium	Loracarbef	Losartan
Lovastatin	Mannitol	Meclofenamate

CREATININE, SERUM

Medications that may increase levels:

Mefenamic acid	Meropenem	Mesalamine
Methicillin	Methotrexate	Methyldopa
Methylprednisolone	Metoprolol	Micardis
Mitomycin	Mitoxantrone	Moexipril
Moxalactam	Mycophenolate	Nalidixic acid
Nandrolone	Naproxen	Neomycin
Netilmicin	Nifedipine	Nilutamide
Nisoldipine	Nitazoxanide	Nitrofurantoin
Norfloxacin	NSAID	Ofloxacin
Olsalazine	Oxacillin	Oxaprozin
Pamidronate	Paromomycin	Pegaspargase
Penicillamine	Penicillin	Pentamidine
Pentostatin	Phenazopyridine	Phosphorus
Piperacillin	Piroxicam	Plicamycin
Prednisone	Propafenone	Propranolol
Quazepam	Quinapril	Radiographic agents
Ramipril	Ranitidine	Risperidone
Salsalate	Sargramostim	Sevoflurane
Sirolimus	Sodium oxybate	Spironolactone
Streptokinase	Streptomycin	Streptozocin
Sulfamethoxazole	Sulfasalazine	Sulfisoxazole
Sulindac	Suprofen	Tacrolimus
Tetracycline	Thiazides	Ticarcillin
Ticlopidine	Timolol	Tobramycin
Tolazoline	Tramadol	Trandolapril
Tretinoin	Triamterene	Triazolam
Trimethoprim	Trimetrexate	Trovafloxacin
Ursodiol	Valsartan	Vancomycin
Vasopressin	Venlafaxine	Vitamin D
Zoledronic acid		

Medications that may decrease levels:

Alprazolam	Amikacin	Ascorbic acid
Atenolol	Cannabis	Captopril
Chlorambucil	Dobutamine	Dopamine
Ibuprofen	Interferon-alfa-2a	Ketoprofen
Lisinopril	Methyldopa	Nicardipine
Prednisone	Quinapril	Terazosin
Triazolam	Tromethamine	Valproic acid
Zidovudine		

CREATININE, URINE

NORMAL VALUES
Men: 14-26 mg/kg/24 hr; 124-230 μmol/kg/24 hr (SI)
Women: 11-20 mg/kg/24 hr; 97-177 μmol/kg/24 hr (SI)

NUTRITIONAL SIGNIFICANCE

Creatinine is formed from creatine, a compound found almost exclusively in muscle tissue. Creatine is synthesized from the amino acids glycine and arginine with addition of a methyl group. It is a high-energy phosphate buffer, maintaining a constant supply of ATP for muscle contraction. Creatinine has no specific biologic function. It is continuously released from the muscle cells and excreted by the kidneys with little reabsorption. When a patient follows a meat-restricted diet, the size of the patient's somatic (muscle) protein pool is directly proportional to the amount of creatinine excreted. The clinical significance is that men generally excrete larger amounts of creatinine than women do and that individuals with greater muscular development excrete larger amounts than those who are less muscular. Total body weight is not proportional to creatinine excretion. Creatinine excretion rate is related to muscle mass in healthy individuals.

The use of urinary creatinine to assess somatic protein status in a healthcare setting in which patients/residents are consuming a mixed diet has its limitations. Creatine is a component of muscle meats. Dietary creatine is converted to creatinine. The body can not distinguish between dietary creatine, which is converted to creatinine, from endogenously produced creatinine. In addition, urinary creatinine can vary significantly

CREATININE, URINE

within individuals, probably because of sweat losses. Urinary creatinine concentration as a biomarker of muscle mass is typically used only in research.

RELATED TESTS: BUN, creatinine

Increased with:
- Acromegaly
- Giantism
- Diabetes mellitus
- Hypothyroidism
- High meat diet
- Creatine supplements

Decreased with:
- Hyperthyroidism
- Anemia
- Muscular dystrophy
- Polymyositis, neurogenic atrophy
- Leukemia
- Advanced renal disease
- Renal Stenosis

Medications that may increase levels:
Aminoglycosides	Ascorbic acid	Cefoxitin
Cephalosporins	Cephalothin	Cimetidine
Cisplatin	Corticosteroids	Fluoxymestrone
Gentamicin	Methotrexate	Methyldopa
Nandrolone	Nitrofurantoin	Nitrofurazone
Oxymetholone	Prednisone	

Medications that may decrease levels:
Anabolic steroids	Captopril	Cephalosporins
Cimetidine	Ketoprofen	Nandrolone
Prednisone	Quinapril	Thiazides
Trimethoprim		

ERYTHROCYTE SEDIMENTATION RATE (ESR)

NORMAL VALUES
Newborn:	0-2 mm/hr
Child:	0-10 mm/hr
Males:	0-15 mm/hr (over 50 yr: 0-20 mm/hr)
Females:	0-20 mm/hr (over 50 yr: 0-30 mm/hr)

NUTRITIONAL SIGNIFICANCE

Sedimentation occurs when RBC aggregate or clump together in a rouleaux formation (stack up in a column-like manner). These changes are due to inflammatory and necrotic processes that alter plasma proteins making the RBC heavier and more likely to settle rapidly. Normally erythrocytes settle slowly and do not form rouleaux.

ESR is the rate at which RBC settle out of anticoagulated blood in one hour. This test is ordered when symptoms are nonspecific. It is used to monitor the course of disease therapy for inflammatory autoimmune diseases such as temporal arteritis or polymyalgia rheumatica. If the patient is being treated with steroids, the ESR will fall with clinical improvement.

RELATED TESTS: ANA, Complement assay, fibrinogen, CRP, RF

Increased with:
- Chronic renal failure
- Gangrene of extremity
- Hyperfibrinogenemia
- Macroglobulinemia
- Collagen diseases
- Hyperthyroidism
- Hypothyroidism
- Heavy-metal poisoning
- Myocardial infarction

ESR Normal (no increase) with:
- Sickle cell anemia
- Spherocytosis
- Hypofibrinogenemia
- Polycythemia vera
- Hereditary spherocytosis
- Acute allergy
- Peptic ulcer
- Congestive heart failure
- Pyruvate kinase deficiency

ERYTHROCYTE SEDIMENTATION RATE (ESR)

Increased with:
- Bacterial infections:
  - pneumonia
  - acute pelvic inflammatory disease
  - syphilis
  - tuberculosis
- Inflammatory diseases:
  - temporal arteritis
  - polymyalgia rheumatica
  - rheumatoid arthritis
  - rheumatic fever
  - acute pelvic inflammatory disease
  - systemic lupus erythematosus
- Cancers
  - multiple myeloma
  - Hodgkin's disease
  - colon
  - lymphoma
  - breast
- Necrotic tissue disease
- Anemias
  - iron deficiency, advanced
  - pernicious anemia, advanced
  - anemia of chronic and inflammatory diseases
- Renal diseases
  - chronic renal failure
  - nephritis, nephrosis
- Toxemia of pregnancy

ESR Normal (no increase) with:
- CRF with heart failure

Erythrocyte Sedimentation Rate (ESR)

Medications that may increase levels:

Anticonvulsants	Aspirin	Carbamazepine
Cephalothin	Cephapirin	Clozapine
Cyclosporine	Dexamethasone	Dextran
Etretinate	Fluvastatin	Hydralazine
Indomethacin	Isotretinoin	Lomefloxacin
Methyldopa	Methysergide	Misoprostol
Ofloxacin	Oral contraceptives	Penicillamine
Procainamide	Propafenone	Quinidine
Sulfamethoxazole	Theophylline	Vitamin A
Zolpidem		

Medications that may decrease levels:

Aspirin	Corticotropin	Cortisone
Cyclophosphamide	Dexamethasone	Gold
Hydroxychloroquine	Leflunomide	Methotrexate
Minocycline	NSAID	Penicillamine
Prednisolone	Prednisone	Quinidine
Sulfasalazine	Tamoxifen	Trimethoprim

FERRITIN

NORMAL VALUES
Newborn :	25-200 ng/mL; 25-200 mcg/L (SI)
< 1 month:	50-200 ng/mL; 50-200 mcg/L (SI)
2-5 mos:	50-200 ng/mL; 50-200 mcg/L (SI)
6 mos-15 yr:	7-142 ng/mL; 7-142 mcg/L (SI)
Adult Males:	12-300 ng/mL; 12-300 mcg/L (SI)
With anemia of chronic disease	< 100 ng/mL; 100 mcg/L (SI)
Adult Females:	10-150 ng/mL; 10-150 mcg/L (SI)
With anemia of chronic disease	< 20 ng/mL; 20 mcg/L (SI)

NUTRITIONAL SIGNIFICANCE

Ferritin is a complex of ferric hydroxide and a protein, apoferritin. It originates in the reticuloendothelial system. Serum ferritin is a test historically used to indicate iron stores. Serum concentrations of ferritin are directly related to iron storage. In individuals with normal iron storage, 1 ng/mL of serum ferritin is approximately 8 mg of stored iron. Ferritin levels in adult males and postmenopausal women are usually significantly higher than in younger females. In one study, levels of ferritin in the upper ranges were highly correlated with increased risk for CAD. It increases in individuals with macrocytic anemia, hemolytic anemia and chronic hepatitis. Ferritin is falsely elevated in neoplasm, alcoholism, uremia, collagen diseases and chronic liver disease. Ferritin stores are also used to monitor iron stores in patients with chronic renal failure. Increased levels are an indicator of iron excess such as hemochromatosis and hemosiderosis.

Ferritin levels can act as an 'acute phase' reactant protein and may be elevated in conditions that do not reflect iron stores

FERRITIN

such as acute inflammation, infections, alcoholism, uremia, chronic liver diseases metastatic cancer, and lymphoma. During inflammatory stress, cytokines impair the production of erythrocytes and reorient iron stores from hemoglobin and serum iron to ferritin. During inflammatory processes IL-1β inhibits the production and release of transferrin while stimulating the synthesis of ferritin. Elevations in ferritin occur 1 to 2 days after the onset of the acute illness and peak at 3 to 5 days. Laboratory test results used to predict the risk of nutritional anemias are not useful in assessing the patient with inflammatory response. If iron deficiency is a co-morbidity, it may not be diagnosed because the level of ferritin would be falsely elevated. Ferritin levels tend to increase with age and in those who eat red meats.

Patients with macrocytic anemias have low hemoglobins and hematocrit, but elevated ferritin. The abnormally large RBC lyse and release iron into the bloodstream. Ferritin production is stimulated to store excess iron. Ferritin values are used in conjunction with hemoglobin, serum iron, TIBC and transferrin to differentiate and classify anemias. Refer to Table 14.

Levels < 10 ng/mL; < 10 mcg/L usually indicated iron deficiency anemia. Decreased levels are associated with iron deficiency anemia and severe protein depletion. A ferritin level of < 10 ng/100 mL suggests iron deficiency anemia. If individual is severely protein depleted, malnutrition may be a contributor to low ferritin levels. Vegetarian tend to have lower ferritin levels.

FERRITIN

Ferritin is not of value in elevating iron stores in individuals with alcoholic related liver disease.

RELATED TESTS: iron levels, TIBC, transferrin, H/H

TABLE 14. Ferritin vs. Serum Fe in Different Conditions

Medical condition	Ferritin	Serum Fe
Hemorrhage, acute	↔	↓
Hemorrhage, chronic	↓	↓
Iron deficiency anemia	↓	↓
Aplastic anemia	↓	↑
Megaloblastic anemia	↑	↓
Pernicious anemia	↑	↓
Hemolytic anemia	↑	↑
Sideroblastic anemia	↑	↑
Thalassemia	↑	↔/↑
Bone marrow neoplasia	↔/↑	↑
Uremia, nephrosis or nephrotic syndrome	↔/↑	↑/↓
Liver diseases	↔/↑	↔/↑

Key: ↔ normal, ↑ increased, ↓ decreased

Increased with:
- Hemochromatosis
- Hemosiderosis
- Collagen vascular diseases
- Hyperthyroidism
- Inflammatory diseases
- Liver disease
  - alcoholic/inflammatory
  - cirrhosis
  - chronic hepatitis

Decreased with:
- Iron deficiency anemia
- Severe protein deficiency
- Hemodialysis

FERRITIN

Increased with:
- Anemias
  - megaloblastic anemia
  - hemolytic anemia
  - thalassemia
  - sideroblastic anemia
  - pernicious anemia
- End stage renal disease
- Cancers
  - Hodgkin's disease
  - breast cancer
  - myoblastic or lymphoblastic leukemia
  - renal cell cancer

Medications that may increase levels:
Ferrous sulfate   Oral contraceptives   Theophylline

Medications that may decrease levels:
Antithyroid therapy   Ascorbic acid   Deferoxamine
Methimazole

FIBRINOGEN (FACTOR I, QUANTITATIVE FIBRINOGEN)

NORMAL VALUES
Newborn: 125-300 mg/dL; 1.25-3 g/L (SI)
Adults: 200-400 mg/dL; 2-4 g/L (SI)

NUTRITIONAL SIGNIFICANCE

Fibrinogen is a polypeptide produced in the liver and is an essential component of the fourth reaction in the coagulation system. It is converted to fibrin by the action of thrombin during the coagulation process. Fibrinogen is also an acute phase reactant protein. It increases sharply during tissue inflammation or tissue necrosis. Elevated levels of fibrinogen have been associated with an increased risk for CAD, stroke, myocardial infarction and peripheral arterial disease. Reduced levels have been reported in patients with liver disease because adequate volumes cannot be synthesized. Lower levels are also observed in malnutrition and disseminated intravascular coagulation (DIC). Patients receiving large volume transfusions will also experience reduced levels of fibrinogen because banked blood does not contain fibrinogen. Diets with a balance of omega-3 and omega-6 fatty acids are associated with reduced levels of fibrogen. Reduced levels of fibrinogen will cause prolonged prothrombin and partial thrombin times. Spontaneous bleeding can occur when values are < 100 mg/dL; 1.0 g/L (SI).

RELATED TESTS: thrombin time, PTT, partial thrombin time, coagulation factor concentration, thrombosis indicators.

FIBRINOGEN (FACTOR I, QUANTITATIVE FIBRINOGEN)

Increased with:
- Acute inflammatory reactions/infections
  - pneumonia
  - rheumatoid arthritis
  - tuberculosis
  - trauma
- Acute MI
- CAD
- Stroke
- Peripheral vascular disease
- Cancers
  - multiple myeloma
  - Hodgkin's disease
- Renal diseases
  - nephrotic syndrome
  - glomerulonephritis
- Smoking
- Pregnancy, eclampsia

Decreased with:
- Congenital afibrinogenemia
- DIC
- Fibrinolysins
- Liver diseases
  - hepatitis
  - cirrhosis
- Advanced carcinoma
- Malnutrition
- Large volume transfusions
- Dysfibrinogenemia

Medications that may increase levels:

Bicalutamide	Chemotherapy	Estropipate
Fluvastatin	Gemfibrozil	Lovastatin
Norethandrolone	Oral contraceptives	Oxandrolone
Oxymetholone	Pyrazinamide	Simvastatin

Medications that may decrease levels:

5-fluorouracil	Anabolic steroids	Anistreplase
Asparaginase	Atenolol	Cefamandole
Clofibrate	Danazol	Dextran
Estrogen/progestin therapy	Factor VIIa	Fenofibrate
Gemfibrozil	Iron	Kanamycin
Lamotrigine	Lovastatin	Medroxyprogesterone
Pegaspargase	Pentoxifylline	Phosphorus
Pravastatin	Prednisone	Raloxifene
Reteplase	Simvastatin	Streptokinase
Sulfisoxazole	Ticlopidine	Valproic acid

FOLATE, SERUM & RED CELL FOLATE (RBC FOLATE)

NORMAL VALUES SERUM
Infants: 14-51 ng/mL; 32-116 nmol/L (SI)
Children: 5-21 ng/mL; 11-48 nmol/L (SI)
Adults: 3-13 ng/mL; 7-30 nmol/L (SI)

NORMAL VALUES RED CELL (RBC FOLATE)
Children: > 160 ng/mL; > 362 nmol/L (SI)
Adults : 140-628 ng/mL; 317-1422 nmol/L(SI)

NUTRITIONAL SIGNIFICANCE

Folic acid (pteroylmonoglutamic acid) and folate (the anion form) are forms of a water-soluble B vitamin. Folic acid is the synthetic form of this vitamin that is found in supplements and fortified foods. Folate functions as a coenzyme in single-carbon transfers in the metabolism of nucleic and amino acids, and is necessary for the synthesis of certain purines and pyrimidines that serve as precursors for DNA. Folate is required for all normal cell division. It is required for normal function of RBC and WBC.

There is a metabolic interrelationship between folate and vitamin B12. A deficiency of either or both nutrients retards DNA synthesis which triggers dyspoiesis or abnormal rate of RBC maturation in the bone marrow. Without adequate vitamin B12, folate becomes trapped in an unusable form, creating a deficiency state at the cellular level even though the dietary intake may be adequate. Vitamin B12 and folate status need to be evaluated concurrently when there are signs of macrocytic anemia.

Folate levels are used to evaluate hemolytic disorders and to detect megaloblastic anemias. In megaloblastic anemia, the

FOLATE, SERUM & RED CELL FOLATE (RBC FOLATE)

abnormally large RBC have a shortened life span because they lyse attempting to enter blood capillaries and they have an impaired oxygen-carrying capacity. Primary causes of megaloblastic anemia include deficient diet, malabsorption syndrome, pregnancy, medication-nutrient interaction, and vitamin B12 deficiency. Some medications are folate antagonists and interfere with nucleic acid synthesis including alcohol, anticonvulsants, antimalarials, aminopterin and methotrexate. Chronic use of antacids or H2 receptor antagonists by patients with inadequate folate intakes are at increased risk for a folate deficiency. Megaloblastic anemia occurs after approximately 4-5 months of folate depletion. Decreased folate levels are associated with megaloblastic anemia, hemolytic anemia, malnutrition, malabsorption syndromes, liver disease and celiac disease. Signs of folic acid deficiency are often subtle. Diarrhea, loss of appetite, and weight loss can occur. Additional signs are weakness, sore tongue, headaches, heart palpitations, irritability and behavioral disorders. Women with folate deficiency who become pregnant are more likely to give birth to low birth weight and premature infants, and infants with neural tube defects. In adults, macrocytic anemia is a sign of advanced folate deficiency. In infants and children, folate deficiency can slow growth rate.

Elevated levels of folate may be seen in pernicious anemia because without sufficient vitamin B12, folate is trapped in an unusable form. The folate test is typically done in conjunction

FOLATE, SERUM & RED CELL FOLATE (RBC FOLATE)

with tests for vitamin B_{12} deficiency to determine if one or both are deficient. If vitamin B12 deficiency presents, treat it first. Folate supplementation will mask the hematological signs of pernicious anemia, while neurological damage continues. The most sensitive measure of folate status is the RBC folate level. Folate is taken up by the developing erythrocyte in the bone marrow and not by the circulating mature erythrocyte during its 120 day lifespan. RBC folate concentration is considered an indicator of long term status.

RELATED TESTS: vitamin B12, Schilling Test, CBC

Increased with:
- Pernicious anemia
- Vegetarianism
- Large blood transfusions
- Blind loop syndrome

Decreased with:
- Folate deficiency
- Megaloblastic anemia
- Hemolytic anemia
- Malnutrition
- Malabsorption syndromes
- Sprue/ Celiac disease
- Crohn's disease
- Ulcerative colitis
- Intestinal resection
- Jejunal bypass procedure
- Liver disease
  - cirrhosis
  - hepatoma
  - alcoholism
- Hypothyroidism
- Carcinomas, metastatic
  - acute leukemia
  - myelofibrosis
- Anorexia nervosa
- Chronic renal failure
- Pregnancy
- Vitamin B6 deficiency
- Infantile hyperthyroidism

FOLATE, SERUM & RED CELL FOLATE (RBC FOLATE)

Medications that may decrease levels:

Acetylsalicylic acid	Allopurinol	Aminopterin
Aminosalicylic acid	Ampicillin	Antacids
Anticonvulsants	Antifungal agents	Aspirin
Barbiturates	Chloramphenicol	Cholestyramine
Colchicine	Cycloserine	Diethylstilbestrol
Erythromycin	Estropipate	Hydrocortisone
Iron	Isoniazid	Levodopa
Lincomycin	Metaxalone	Metformin
Methacholine	Methenamine	Methotrexate
Nitrofurantoin	Oral contraceptives	Penicillin
Pentamidine	Phenobarbital	Phenytoin
Primidone	Pyrimethamine	Rifampin
Sulfamethoxazole	Sulfasalazine	Sulfisoxazole
Tetracycline	Triamterene	Trimethoprim

GLUCOSE, BLOOD

NORMAL VALUES
Cord:	45-96 mg/dL; 2.5-5.3 mmol/L (SI)
Premature Infant:	20-60 mg/dL; 1.1-3.3 mmol/L (SI)
Neonate:	30-60 mg/dL; 1.7-3.3 mmol/L (SI)
Infant:	40-90 mg/dL; 2.2-5.0 mmol/L (SI)
Child < 2 yr:	60-100 mg/dL; 3.3-5.5 mmol/L (SI)

Child > 2yr to Adult:
Fasting*	70-100 mg/dL; 3.9-5.5 mmol/L (SI)
Casual**	< 200 mg/dL; < 11.1 mmol/L (SI)
Elderly:	increased slightly after age 50

* fasting- no caloric intake for at least 8 hr
** casual- any time of day regardless of food intake

NUTRITIONAL SIGNIFICANCE

Glucose is formed from the digestion of carbohydrate and the conversion of glycogen by the liver. Levels are regulated by insulin and glucagon. When food is eaten, the beta cells of the pancreas secrete insulin, which increases cellular membrane permeability to glucose. Driving glucose into the cells requires insulin and insulin receptors. Glucose is metabolized into glycogen, amino acids and fatty acids. Adrenocorticosteroid, adrenocorticotropic hormone, epinephrine and thyroxine can also affect glucose metabolism.

When food is not eaten for an extended period of time the blood glucose drops, the pancreas secretes glucagon, which in turn acts on the liver to convert glycogen into glucose. The result is the blood glucose levels return to normal ranges.

Individuals experiencing severe stress from injury, burns or surgery have elevated glucose levels because the physiological

GLUCOSE, BLOOD

stress stimulates the catecholamine release. This in turn stimulates glucagon secretion which causes hyperglycemia. Inflammatory stress also triggers the release of proinflammatory cytokines which increase insulin resistance in muscles resulting in hyperglycemia.

When the pancreas fails to secrete insulin in adequate amounts or is delayed in responding to food intake, the blood glucose will continue to increase. Once renal threshold is reached (around 180 mg/dL; 10 mmol/L), the kidneys attempt to decrease the abnormally high blood glucose through increased diuresis. Critical values for hyperglycemia in adults are > 400 mg/dL; 22 mmol/L and in the newborn are >300 mg/dL; 17 mmol/L.

When the liver fails to secrete glucagon in response to low blood glucose the levels continue to fall. This process indicates that either the body is unable to convert glycogen to glucose or the glycogen stores are depleted. Critical values for hypoglycemia in adult males are < 50 mg/dL; 2.8 mmol/L, adult females, children and infants are < 40 mg/dL; 2.2 mmol/L and in newborn < 30 mg/dL; 1.7 mmol/L.

Serum glucose level is a test used to diagnose many metabolic diseases. Levels must be evaluated at different times of day for an accurate diagnosis. For example, a blood glucose level of 132 mg/dL may be abnormal in a fasting state, but within normal limits if the person has just finished a meal. Non-nutritional factors may elevate fasting blood glucose including

GLUCOSE, BLOOD

stress, infection, caffeine and smoking. A careful review of the health history of the patient and clear instructions for the test are essential to lessen the effects of non-nutritional factors.

The most common diagnosis associated with elevated blood glucose is diabetes mellitus. A fasting blood glucose test is performed on serum or plasma rather than whole blood. Values will vary from the whole blood glucose tests performed on capillary blood using the fingerstick method. Laboratory values are likely 10-15 percent higher than capillary values. The diagnosis of diabetes is made using a variety of criteria including both physical assessment and laboratory assessment of blood glucose control. Testing is recommended to detect pre-diabetes (impaired glucose tolerance) and type 2 diabetes in asymptomatic patients with BMI > 25 and who have one or more risk factors for diabetes. Refer to Standards of Medical Care in Diabetes (2009, 2010) for details. Tables 15-16 include screening criteria for diabetes.

TABLE 15. Interpretation of FPG for DM Screening

Criteria using FBG	Interpretation
FPG <100 mg/dL; 5.5 mmol/L	normal fasting glucose
FPG ≥100 mg/dL < 125 mg/dL; 5.51 – 6.9 mmol/L	IFG or IGT or pre-diabetes
FPG ≥126 mg/dL; 7 mmol/L	provisional diagnosis of diabetes

Fasting blood glucose testing requires the individual to not eat for 8 hr before the test and not take their usual insulin or oral hypoglycemic agent. In individuals with insulin dependent diabetes the test indicates the adequacy of overnight insulinization and can be used to adjust insulin dosage. In individuals with

GLUCOSE, BLOOD

NIDDM the test measures the endogenous overnight insulin secretion. The results may suggest the need for tighter metabolic control.

American Association for Clinical Endocrinology and American Diabetes Association issued a consensus statement on inpatient glycemic control signalling a shift in practice from very tight glucose control to a more moderate level of control in hospitalized individuals with diabetes. The current recommendation is to maintain a goal of 110-180 mg/dL for critically ill patients and a goal of < 140 mg/dL premeal and < 180 mg/dL random blood glucose for the non-critically ill(2009).

TABLE 16. DM Diagnostic Criteria for Non-pregnant Adults

Criteria using fasting blood glucose
FPG $\geq$ 126 mg/dL; 7.0 mmol/L after an 8 hour fast
Signs & symptoms of diabetes plus casual plasma glucose concentration $\geq$ 200 mg/dL; 11 mmol/L
2hr PG $\geq$ 200 mg/dL; 11 mmol/L during OGTT (75 gm load)
Criteria using Hemoglobin A1C
HbA1C 6.5% or higher (Refer to subsequent section)

Risk assessment for gestational diabetes mellitus (GDM) is usually done at the first prenatal visit. Women at very high risk for GDM should be screened for diabetes as soon as possible. Criteria for the very high risk includes severe obesity, prior history of GDM, history of large-for gestational-age infant, glucosuria, PCOS, and strong family history type 2 diabetes. Screening for all women

GLUCOSE, BLOOD

of greater than low risk for GDM are done between 24-28 weeks gestation. Low risk status is defined as women who meet all these characteristics; less than 25 yr old, weight normal before pregnancy, member of ethnic group with low prevalence of diabetes, no first-degree relatives with diabetes, no history of abnormal glucose tolerance, no history of poor obstetrical outcome. Refer to post prandial glucose and oral glucose tolerance test for more information on diagnostic criteria for GDM.

Blood glucose levels > 300 mg/dL; 16.6 mmol/L are associated with falsely low serum sodium values. Serum sodium levels are usually low for one of three reasons:

- The osmotically active glucose draws water from cells into intravascular space creating a dilution effect.
- Severe hypertriglyceridemia plus the metabolic decompensation may displace some of the aqueous component of the blood and sodium is only found in the aqueous component.
- Dehydration stimulates increased water retention creating a dilution effect.

Consult laboratory for formulas to estimate true serum sodium levels.

RELATED TESTS: diabetes mellitus autoantibody panel, glucose, urine, A1C, GTT, PPG, glucagon, insulin assay

Increased with:
- Chronic liver disease
- Trauma
- Caffeine

Decreased with:
- Alcoholism
- Starvation
- Malabsorption

GLUCOSE, BLOOD

Increased with:
- Acromegaly
- Gigantism
- Dehydration
- CVA
- Pregnancy
- Convulsions
- Obesity
- Cystic fibrosis DM
- Diabetes
- General anesthesia
- Hyperthyroidism
- Stress
- Cushing's syndrome
- Pituitary adenoma
- Acute pancreatitis
- Adenoma of pancreas
- Hemochromatosis
- Myocardial infarction
- Acute stress response
- Pheochromocytoma
- Chronic renal failure
- Glucagonoma
- Wernicke's encephalopathy
- Heavy smoking

Decreased with:
- Endocrine disorders
  - Addison's disease
  - hypothyroidism
  - hypopituitarism
  - ACTH deficiency
- Reactive hypoglycemia
- Enzyme disorders:
  - Von Gierke's disease
  - galactosemia
  - maple syrup urine disease
  - fructose intolerance
- Liver disease:
  - hepatitis
  - cirrhosis
  - poisoning
  - metastatic tumor
- Pancreatic disorders:
  - glucagon deficiency
  - islet cell carcinoma
- Insulin overdose
- Insulinoma
- Water overload
- Hematocrit > 55%
- Premature infant of GDM mother
- Extrapancreatic stomach tumors
- Intense exercise
- Toxic doses of, aspirin salicylates, acetaminophen

GLUCOSE, BLOOD

Medications that may increase levels (can lead to false positive value):

Abacavir	Acebutolol	Acetaminophen
Acetazolamide	Adenosine	Albuterol
Alcohol	Aldesleukin	Aminophylline
Aminosalicylic acid	Amiodarone	Amitriptyline
Amoxapine	Amphotericin B	Ampicillin/Sulbactam
Antidepressants	Aripiprazole	Asparaginase
Aspirin	Atazanavir	Atenolol
Atropine	Azathioprine	Azithromycin

Medications that may increase levels (can lead to false positive value):

Baclofen	Basiliximab	Beclomethasone
Benazepril	Beta adrenergic blockers	Betamethasone
Betaxolol	Bicalutamide	Bisoprolol
Budesonide	Calcitonin	Candesartan
Cannabis	Captopril	Carvedilol
Cefdinir	Cefotaxime	Cefpodoxime
Cefuroxime	Chloramphenicol	Chlorothiazide
Chlorpromazine	Chlorthalidone	Cholestyramine
Cidofovir	Clofibrate	Clonidine
Clozapine	Colchicine	Corticosteroids
Corticotropin	Cortisone	Cyclobenzaprine
Cyclophosphamide	Cyclosporine	Daclizumab
Danazol	Desipramine	Dexamethasone
Dextran	Dextroamphetamine	Dextrose IV infusions
Dextrothyroxine	Diazoxide	Diclofenac
Didanosine	Diethylstilbestrol	Diltiazem
Dimercaprol	Diphenoxylate	Dobutamine
Donepezil	Dopamine	Doxepin
Doxorubicin	Enalapril	Enfuvirtide
Ephedra	Ephedrine	Epinephrine
Escitalopram	Estrogens	Estropipate
Ethacrynic acid	Ethionamide	Etretinate
Felbamate	Felodipine	Fenofibrate
Fludrocortisone	Fluoxymesterone	Fluvoxamine
Fosamprenavir	Foscarnet	Fosinopril
Fosphenytoin	Furosemide	Ganciclovir
Gemfibrozil	Glimepiride	Glucagon
Glucosamine	Goserelin	Growth hormone

GLUCOSE, BLOOD

Medications that may increase levels (can lead to false positive value):

Haloperidol	Hydralazine	Hydrochlorothiazide
Hydroflumethiazide	Imipramine	Indapamide
Indinavir	Indomethacin	Interferon α-2a
Interferon γ-1b	Irinotecan	Iron
Isoniazid	Isoproterenol	Isotretinoin
Ketoprofen	Labetalol	Lactose
Lansoprazole	Leuprolide	Levalbuterol
Levodopa	Levodopa/carbidopa	Levofloxacin
Levonorgestrel	Liothyronine	Lisinopril
Lithium	Loperamide	Maprotiline
Medroxyprogesterone	Mefenamic acid	Megestrol
Meperidine	Mercaptopurine	Methandrostenolone
Methimazole	Methyclothiazide	Methyldopa
Methylprednisolone	Metolazone	Metoprolol
Metronidazole	Mirtazapine	Molindone
Morphine	Mycophenolate	Nabumetone
Nalidixic acid	Naproxen	Nelfinavir
Niacin	Niacinamide	Nicotinic Acid
Nifedipine	Nilutamide	Nisoldipine
Nitrofurantoin	Norethindrone	Norfloxacin
Nortriptyline	Octreotide	Ofloxacin
Olanzapine	Oral contraceptives	Oxazepam
Palonosetron	Pancreozymin	Paraldehyde
Paroxetine	Pegaptanib	Pegaspargase
Pentamidine	Pergolide	Perindopril
Perphenazine	Phenazopyridine	Phenelzine
Phenothiazine	Phenylephrine	Phenytoin
Pindolol	Piroxicam	Polythiazide
Pravastatin	Prazosin	Prednisone
Probenecid	Propafenone	Propranolol
Propylthiouracil	Protriptyline	Quinapril
Quinethazone	Ramipril	Reserpine
Rifampin	Riluzole	Risperidone
Ritonavir	Saquinavir	Sargramostim
Sildenafil	Sodium oxybate	Somatostatin
Spironolactone	Streptomycin	Streptozocin
Sulfisoxazole	Sulindac	Sumatriptan
Tacrine	Tacrolimus	Terbutaline
Tetracycline	Theophylline	Thiabendazole
Thiazides	Thiothixene	

GLUCOSE, BLOOD

Medications that may increase levels (can lead to false positive value):

Thyroid	Timolol	Tolbutamide
Tolcapone	Triamcinolone	Triamterene
Triazolam	Trichlormethiazide	Trifluoperazine
Trimethoprim	Trimetrexate	Trimipramine
Ursodiol	Valproic acid	Venlafaxine
Verapamil	Vidarabine	Vitamin C/Ascorbic Acid
Zalcitabine	Zidovudine	Ziprasidone
Zolmitriptan	Zolpidem	

Medications that may decrease levels (can lead to false negative value):

Acarbose	Acetaminophen	Acetaminophen/ codeine
Acetazolamide	Acetohexamide	Aldesleukin
Allopurinol	Amphetamine	Anabolic steroids
Aspirin	Atenolol	Atropine
Basiliximab	Benazepril	Butalbital/ caffeine acetaminophen/codeine
Butalbital/ caffeine acetaminophen	Calcium gluconate	Cannabinol
Captopril	Carvedilol	Cefdinir
Cefpodoxime	Cefuroxime	Chloramphenicol
Chloroquine	Chlorpromazine	Chlorpropamide
Cholestyramine	Cimetidine	Ciprofloxacin
Clofibrate	Desipramine	Dextroamphetamine
Diazepam	Diazoxide	Diltiazem
Dimercaprol	Disopyramide	Doxazosin
Doxepin	Doxorubicin	Duloxetine
Enalapril	Erythromycin	Ethacrynic acid
Etretinate	Felbamate	Fenfluramine
Fenofibrate	Flucytosine	Fluoxymesterone
Flurazepam	Fluvoxamine	Foscarnet
Fosinopril	Furosemide	Ganciclovir
Gemfibrozil	Glimepiride	Glipizide
Glucosamine	Glyburide	GCSF
Green tea	Guanethidine	Guar
Haloperidol	Hydralazine	Hydrocodone/ acetaminophen

GLUCOSE, BLOOD

Medications that may decrease levels (can lead to false negative value):

Imipramine	Indomethacin	Insulin
Interferon β 1 b	Isocarboxazid	Isoniazid
Lansoprazole	Leuprolide	Levodopa
Levofloxacin	Lisinopril	Lomefloxacin
MAO inhibitors	Maprotiline	Megestrol
Metformin	Methyldopa	Methyltestosterone
Metoprolol	Metronidazole	Midazolam
Miglitol	Mycophenolate	Nadolol
Nandrolone	Nefazodone	Nelfinavir
Niacin	Nifedipine	Norethindrone
Norfloxacin	Nortriptyline	Octreotide
Ofloxacin	Oxandrolone	Oxycodone/ acetaminophen
Oxymetholone	Oxytetracycline	Pargyline
Paroxetine	Pegaspargase	Penicillamine
Pentamidine	Pergolide	Perindopril
Perphenazine	Phenazopyridine	Phentolamine
Phosphorus	Pioglitazone	Piroxicam
Prazosin	Prednisone	Probenecid
Progesterone	Promethazine	Propoxyphene
Propranolol	Protriptyline	Quinapril
Quinine	Ramipril	Repaglinide
Rosiglitazone	Saquinavir	Selegiline
Sildenafil	Simvastatin	Somatostatin
St. John's Wort	Sulfamethoxazole	Sulfisoxazole
Sumatriptan	Terazosin	Terbutaline
Tetracycline	Thiabendazole	Tolazamide
Tolbutamide	Trastuzumab	Trimethoprim
Trimipramine	Troglitazone	Tromethamine
Valproic acid	Verapamil	Vitamin C/Ascorbic Acid

GLUCOSE, BLOOD, POST PRANDIAL (PPG)

NORMAL VALUES

0-50 yr:	< 140 mg/dL; < 7.8 mmol/dL (SI)
50-60 yr:	< 150 mg/dL; < 8.4 mmol/dL (SI)
60 yr +:	< 160 mg/dL; < 8.9 mmol/dL (SI)
1 hr glucose screen for GDM	< 140 mg/dL; < 7.8 mmol/dL (SI)

NUTRITIONAL SIGNIFICANCE

The post prandial glucose test is a screening test for diabetes mellitus. A meal serves as a glucose challenge to evaluate the body's ability to metabolize glucose. Insulin is normally secreted after a meal in response to elevations in blood glucose, causing the levels to return to normal within 2 hours. In patients with diabetes, the glucose levels usually remain elevated 2 hours after a meal. If the results are > 140 mg/dL; 7.8 mmol/L and < 200 mg/dL; 11 mmol/L, an oral glucose tolerance test (OGTT) may be ordered. If the results are > 200 mg/dL; 11 mmol/L, the diagnosis of diabetes is confirmed. Glycosylated hemoglobin is not used to diagnosis gestational diabetes (GDM) because changes in red cell turnover make the A1C assay problematic.

TABLE 17. Diagnostic Criteria for DM using PPG

Criteria using OGTT	Interpretation
2 hr postload glucose* (2h PPG**) < 140 mg/dL; 7.8 mmol/L	normal PPG
2 hr PPG ≥ 140 and < 200 mg/dL; 7.8-11 mmol/L and < 11mmol/L	IFG or IGT or pre-diabetes
2 hr PPG ≥ 200 mg/dL; 11 mmol/L	provisional dx DM

* glucose load containing equivalent of 75 g anhydrous glucose dissolved in water
IFG-impaired fasting glucose, IGT- impaired glucose tolerance, PPG-postprandial glucose

GLUCOSE, BLOOD, POST PRANDIAL (PPG)

The Standards of Medical Care in Diabetes (2009) recommend diagnostic criteria for detecting GDM as noted in Table 18. GDM affects 3-8 percent of all pregnant women. About 50 percent of these women will develop diabetes later in life. The identification and treatment of gestational diabetes may reduce the risk for several adverse perinatal outcomes.

TABLE 18. Diagnostic Criteria for GDM

Two-Step Approach	Interpretation
Step 1. Plasma or serum glucose 1 hr after 50 g oral glucose load	> or = to 140 mg/dL: 7.8 mmol/L identified about 80% of women with GDM **OR** > or = to 130 mg/dL; 7.2 mmol/L identified about 90% of women with GDM
Step 2. For those that exceed threshold for 50g screening: 100 g oral glucose load	2+ of following plasma glucose must be found: fasting:> or = to 95 mg/dL; 5.3 mmol/L 1 hr: > or = to 180 mg/dL; 10 mmol/L 2 hr: > or = to 155 mg/dL; 8.6 mmol/L 3 hr: > or = to 140 mg/dL; 7.8 mmol/L
One-Step Approach	**Interpretation**
Step 1. 100 g oral glucose load after 8 hr fast	2+ of following plasma glucose must be found: fasting:> or = to 95 mg/dL; 5.3 mmol/L 1 hr: > or = to 180 mg/dL; 10 mmol/L 2 hr: > or = to 155 mg/dL; 8.6 mmol/L 3 hr: > or = to 140 mg/dL; 7.8 mmol/L

RELATED TESTS: FBG, glucose, urine, A1C, GTT

GLUCOSE, BLOOD, POST PRANDIAL (PPG)

Increased with:
- Acromegaly
- Acute stress response
- Chronic renal failure
- Corticosteroid therapy
- Diabetes mellitus
- Diuretic therapy
- Extensive liver disease
- Gestational diabetes
- Malnutrition
- Cushing's syndrome
- Hyperthyroidism
- Pheochromocytoma
- Glucagonoma

Decreased with:
- Addison's disease
- Hypopituitarism
- Hypothyroidism
- Insulin overdose
- Malabsorption
- Maldigestion
- Insulinoma

Medications that may increase levels:

Refer to Glucose, Blood section.

Medications that may decrease levels:

Refer to Glucose, Blood section.

Glucose Tolerance Test, Oral (GTT)

Normal Values
Fasting:	70-100 mg/dL; < 5.5 mmol/L (SI)
30 Minutes:	<200 mg/dL; < 11.1 mmol/L (SI)
1 hr:	<200 mg/dL; < 11.1 mmol/L (SI)
2 hr:	<140 mg/dL; < 7.8 mmol/L (SI)
3 hr:	70-115 mg/dL; < 6.4 mmol/L (SI)
4 hr:	70-115 mg/dL; < 6.4 mmol/L (SI)

Nutritional Significance

The Standards for Diabetes Care (2009) and subsequent addendum (2010) to the recommendations identify four different methodologies for diagnosis of diabetes. A 2 hour oral GTT is one of the methodologies. For some individuals, more extensive testing is recommended. The 4 hour oral GTT evaluates the patient's ability to tolerate a standard oral glucose load (75 gm CHO) at five time intervals. Blood levels are checked at 30 minutes, 1 hour, 2 hours, 3 hours and 4 hours after administration of the oral glucose load. In addition to blood, urine is tested to determine if renal threshold is reached.

Individuals with an appropriate insulin response are able to tolerate the dose of glucose easily. Individuals with insulin dependent or non-insulin dependent diabetes will not be able to tolerate the standard oral glucose load. Serum glucose levels will remain greatly elevated from 1 to 5 hours. Once renal threshold is reached, the urine will test positive for glucose.

Glucose intolerance may occur in patients with abnormal secretions of hormones that have an ancillary affect on glucose. For example, Cushing's syndrome, pheochromocytoma,

GLUCOSE TOLERANCE TEST, ORAL (GTT)

acromegaly, aldosteronism and hyperthyroidism all exhibit glucose intolerance. Individuals with chronic renal failure, acute pancreatitis, myxedema, type IV lipoproteinemia, infection or cirrhosis may have an abnormal oral GTT. Reactive hypoglycemia can be evaluated using the oral GTT. The drop in blood glucose may occur up to five hours after the initial glucose load.

The Standards of Medical Care in Diabetes (2009) recommend diagnostic criteria for detecting gestational diabetes using two different approaches. Diagnostic criteria using oral GTT is noted in Table 19. Women with glucose levels > 140 mg/dL; 7.8 mmol/L should be retested 6 weeks or more after delivery.

TABLE 19. Diagnostic Criteria for GDM using GTT

Approach	Interpretation
100 g oral glucose load after 8 hr fast	2+ of following plasma glucose must be found: fasting:> or = to 95 mg/dL; 5.3 mmol/L 1 hr: > or = to 180 mg/dL; 10 mmol/L 2 hr: > or = to 155 mg/dL; 8.6 mmol/L 3 hr: > or = to 140 mg/dL; 7.8 mmol/L

In patients with a prior gastrectomy, weight loss surgery, short bowel syndrome or a malabsorption syndrome, the oral glucose load on the oral GTT is intolerable. In these individuals an intravenous glucose tolerance test (IV-GTT) is used. The values for the IV-GTT differ slightly from the oral GTT because IV glucose is absorbed faster.

GLUCOSE TOLERANCE TEST, ORAL (GTT)

The oral GTT is contraindicated for persons under significant emotional stress from recent surgery or with concurrent infections. Stress, infections and caffeine can cause an increased blood glucose level. Smoking during the testing period can stimulate glucose due to the nicotine. Exercising during the test will decrease the blood glucose levels if insulin is present. However, when insulin is absent exercise will dramatically increase the blood glucose levels.

RELATED TESTS: FBG, glucose, urine, A1C, PPG

Increased with (glucose rises and does not fall to normal levels)**:**

- Acromegaly
- Acute pancreatitis
- Acute stress response
- Chronic renal failure
- CNS lesions
- Corticosteroid therapy
- Cushing's syndrome
- Diabetes mellitus
- Diuretic therapy
- Gestational diabetes
- Glucagonoma
- Hemochromatosis
- Hyperlipidemia type III, IV, V
- Hyperthyroidism
- ↑ epinephrine levels
- Infection
- Myxedema
- Pancreatic cancer

Decreased with (glucose does not increase or may decrease to hypoglycemic levels **):**

- Pancreatic islet cell hyperplasia or tumor
- Malabsorption
  - sprue
  - Celiac disease
  - Whipple's disease
- Hypoparathyroidism
- Addison's disease
- Liver disease
- Hypopituitarism
- Hypothyroidism

LABORATORY ASSESSMENT OF NUTRITIONAL STATUS:
BRIDGING THEORY & PRACTICE

GLUCOSE TOLERANCE TEST, ORAL (GTT)

Increased with (glucose rises and does not fall to normal levels)**:**
- Pheochromocytoma
- Post gastrectomy
- Reactive hypoglycemia
- Severe liver disease
- Smoking
- Somogyi response to hypoglycemia
- Stress
- von Gierke's disease

Medications that may increase levels:

Refer to Glucose, Blood section.

Medications that may decrease levels:

Refer to Glucose, Blood section.

GLUCOSE, URINE

NORMAL VALUES
Random specimen: Negative
24 hour specimen: <0.5 mg/d or <2.78 mmol/d (SI)

NUTRITIONAL SIGNIFICANCE
Glucose is filtered from the blood by the glomeruli of the kidney. In the non-diabetic, all of the glucose is resorbed in the proximal renal tubules. Urine glucose is part of a routine urinalysis and serves as a screening test for diabetes mellitus. The blood level at which tubular reabsorption stops is called renal threshold. When blood glucose levels reach between 160-180 mg/dL; 9-10 mmol/L the glucose begins to spill over into the urine. Urine glucose levels > 1000 mg/dL; > 55 mmol/L or 4+ are critical values.

Glucose in the urine is not always an indicator of a medical problem. For example, glycosuria can occur after eating a high-carbohydrate meal or after receiving dextrose IV infusions. In the non-diabetic, glycosuria can occur with a normal serum glucose level if kidney disease affects the renal tubule. In this case, the renal threshold for glucose becomes abnormally low and glucose spills into the urine. Also, patients with acute severe physical stress or injury may have transient glycosuria caused by normal compensatory endocrine-mediated responses.

RELATED TESTS: FBS, A1C, PPG, glucagon, insulin assay

Increased with:
- Diabetes mellitus
- Infection
- Drug therapy

GLUCOSE, URINE

Increased with:
- Endocrine disorders:
  - thyrotoxicosis
  - Cushing's syndrome
  - acromegaly
- Severe stress:
  - trauma
  - surgery
- Pregnancy
- Low renal threshold
- Glycosuria
- Fanconi syndrome
- Increased cranial pressure
- Nephrotoxic chemicals
- Liver & pancreatic disease
- CNS disorders
  - brain injury
  - CVA

Medications that may increase levels:

Acetazolamide	Aminosalicylic acid	Ampicillin
Ascorbic acid	Asparaginase	Aspirin
Azlocillin	Benzthiazide	Bismuth subsalicylate
Bupropion	Captopril	Carbamazepine
Carbenicillin	Carvedilol	Cefaclor
Cefamandole	Cefazolin	Cefdinir

Medications that may increase levels:

Cefepime	Cefixime	Cefoperazone
Cefuroxime	Cephalexin	Cephalosporin
Chlorothiazide	Chlorpheniramine	Chlorpromazine
Chlorthalidone	Cidofovir	Corticosteroids
Corticotropin	Cyclobenzaprine	Cyclophosphamide
Dexamethasone	Dextroamphetamine	Diazoxide
Doxorubicin	Enalapril	Ephedrine
Ethacrynic acid	Ether	Ethionamide
Etretinate	Fludrocortisone	Foscarnet

Glucose, Urine

Medications that may increase levels:

Furazolidone	Furosemide	Gabapentin
Histrelin	Hydrochlorothiazide	Ifosfamide
Indomethacin	Isoniazid	Lithium
Methyclothiazide	Metolazone	Mirtazapine
Misoprostol	Nalidixic acid	Naproxen
Niacin	Nitrofurantoin	Norfloxacin
Ofloxacin	Omeprazole	Penicillin
Perphenazine	Phenazopyridine	Phenothiazine
Phenytoin	Piperacillin	Polythiazide
Probenecid	Quinethazone	Reserpine
Ritodrine	Sevoflurane	Somatropin
Streptomycin	Sulfonamide	Tacrine
Tetracycline	Theophylline	Thiazides
Thiothixene	Ticarcillin	Timolol
Triamcinolone	Venlafaxine	

Medications that may decrease levels:

Acarbose	Ampicillin	Ascorbic acid
Aspirin	Bisacodyl	Chloral hydrate
Cholestyramine	Dextrothyroxine	Diazepam
Diazoxide	Digoxin	Estrogens
Ferrous sulfate	Flurazepam	Furosemide
Hydroquinone	Insulin	Isoniazid
Levodopa	Lithium	Nafcillin
Nalidixic acid	Nicotinic acid	Oxytetracycline
Phenazopyridine	Phenobarbital	Radiographic agents
Secobarbital	Tetracycline	Vitamin supplements

GLUCOSE-6-PHOSPHATE DEHYDROGENASE (G-6-PD)

NORMAL VALUES
Children: 6.4-15.6 IU/g Hb; 0.11-0.26 nkat/g Hb (SI)
Adults: 8.6-18.6 IU/g Hb; 0.14-0.31 nkat/g Hb (SI)
Newborns: values up to 50% higher than adults

Some labs report data in U/ml RBC. To convert U/g Hb to U/ml RBCs: U/g Hb X 0.34= U/mL of RBC.

NUTRITIONAL SIGNIFICANCE

      The G-6-PD enzyme catalyzes the oxidation of glucose-6-phosphate to 6-phosphogluconate. At the same time, it also reduces the oxidized form of nicotinamide adenine dinucleotide phosphate (NADP+) to nicotinamide adenine dinucleotide phosphate (NADPH). NADPH, a required cofactor in many biosynthetic reactions, maintains glutathione in its reduced form. Reduced glutathione acts as a scavenger for dangerous oxidative metabolites in the cell. With the help of the enzyme glutathione peroxidase, reduced glutathione also converts harmful hydrogen peroxide to water. RBC rely heavily upon G-6-PD activity because it is the only source of NADPH that protects the cells against oxidative stresses.

      G-6-PD deficiency is a disease that primarily affects men of all races. The highest prevalence is among persons of African, Asian or Mediterranean descent. Severity varies significantly between racial groups because of different variants of the enzyme. Individuals with the disorder are not normally anemic and display no evidence of the disease until the RBC are exposed to an oxidant or stress. Infections, acidosis, consumption of fava beans or

GLUCOSE-6-PHOSPHATE DEHYDROGENASE (G-6-PD)

exposure to certain medications will trigger a rapid hemolysis of erythrocytes. Ultimately, this hemolysis leads to anemia -- either acute hemolytic or a chronic spherocytic type. The episodes of anemia are usually brief, because newly produced RBC have normal G-6-PD activity.

Oxidizing medications such as antimalarials, sulfa, aspirin, phenacetin, antipyretics, quinidine, sulfonamides, thiazide diuretics, tolbutamide and others may cause erythrocyte destruction and hemolysis. Hemolysis can occur between the first and fourth day following ingestion of medication. Infections and acidosis can exacerbate a hemolytic process in these patients.

RELATED TESTS: FBG, glycosylated hemoglobin, GTT

Increased with:
- Pernicious anemia
- Megaloblastic anemia
- Chronic blood loss
- Viral hepatitis
- Hepatic coma
- Myocardial infarction
- Hyperthyroidism

Decreased with:
- G-6-PD deficiency
- Hemolytic anemia
- Unusual nonspherocytic anemia
- Nonimmunologic hemolytic disease of newborn

Medications that Precipitate Hemolysis in G-6-PD Deficient Patients

Acetanilid	Antimalarials	Antipyretics
Ascorbic acid	Aspirin	Dapsone
Methylene blue	Nalidixic acid	Nitrofurantoin
Phenacetin	Phenazopyridine	Primaquine
Quinidine	Sulfa	Sulfonamides
Thiazide diuretics	Tolbutamide	Vitamin K

GLYCOSYLATED HEMOGLOBIN (A1C)

NORMAL VALUES

Non-diabetic Child:	2.2% to 4.8%
Non-diabetic Adult:	2.2% to 4.8%
Good diabetic control:	2.5% - 5.9%
Fair diabetic control:	> 6 % < 8%%
Poor diabetic control:	> 8%

NUTRITIONAL SIGNIFICANCE

Glycosylated hemoglobin (A1C) is a test which provides an accurate 2-3-month index of average blood glucose levels. It has been added as a diagnostic criterion for the diagnosis of diabetes mellitus (2010). Refer to Table 20. While there is no single lab test related to hyperglycemia that is considered the 'gold standard' to predict risk for microvascular or macrovascular disease, A1C is used to monitor chronic glycemia and the effectiveness of diabetes treatment.

TABLE 20. Diagnostic Criteria for DM using A1C

Criteria	Interpretation
A1C > 6.5%	Confirm with repeat A1C unless plasma glucose > 200 mg/dL; 11 mmol/L

A small percentage of RBC will bind to the glucose in the bloodstream. The process is called glycosylation. It is a permanent bond through the life of the RBC (100-120 day life span). The percent of glycohemoglobin in the blood is directly related to the average blood glucose levels. Remember that RBC are constantly being destroyed and new ones are being formed. The A1C value reflects the average blood glucose for 2-3 months

Glycosylated Hemoglobin (A1C)

prior to the test. It does not reflect more recent changes in glucose levels (e.g. 15-20 days). If the patient has had greatly fluctuating blood glucose levels (<50 mg/dL and >200 mg/dL) the test will reflect both highs and lows. In other words, a person in poor control may have relatively good A1C values when in fact the blood glucose control has been poor.

In adults, approximately 98 percent of the hemoglobin is stored in RBC. Glycohemoglobin is seen in approximately 4-6 percent of the total hemoglobin molecules in persons with normal blood glucose control. These molecules are classified as HbA1a, HbA1b and HbA1c. The HbA1c is usually measured because it combines most strongly with glucose. However, some labs measure HbA1. These values are usually 2-4 percent higher than the HbA1c component. Using the cation exchange test methodology normal ranges for HbA1 are 5.5 - 8.5 percent. A1C is a valuable test because the sample can be drawn at any time. In addition, recent food intake, exercise, stress, hypoglycemic agents or patient cooperation does not affect the values. It is used to evaluate the success of diabetic therapy, especially when new strategies for care are implemented. A1C has been used to determine the duration of hyperglycemia in newly diagnosed diabetics as well as those with impaired glucose tolerance. It is helpful to differentiate between short-term hyperglycemia in non-diabetics under stress or had a myocardial infarction and diabetes mellitus. A1C is an additional tool for

GLYCOSYLATED HEMOGLOBIN (A1C)

providing positive feedback to patients. A1C is not used as a diagnostic criterion for GDM because changes in red cell turnover make the A1C assay problematic.

A1C can be correlated accurately with the daily mean plasma glucose (MPG) level or average blood glucose level throughout the day using this formula:

$$MPG = (35.6 \times A1C) - 77.3$$

Refer to Table 21 for approximate MPG.

TABLE 21. Approximate Correlation Between A1C & MPG*

A1C (%)	MPG mg/dL	Interpretation
4	65	Non-diabetic range
5	100	Non-diabetic range
6	135	Non-diabetic range
7	170	ADA target range
8	205	Action needed

* adapted from Pagana & Pagana (2009) *Mosby's Manual of Diagnostic Laboratory Tests*. St. Louis: Mosby.

RELATED TESTS: FBG, glucose, urine, PPG, GTT, glucagon, insulin assay

Increased with:
- Newly diagnosed or poorly controlled diabetes
- Impaired glucose tolerance
- Hyperglycemia
- Pregnancy
- Fe deficiency anemia
- Hemodialysis
- Alcohol toxicity

Decreased with:
- Hemolytic anemia (Sickle Cell due to increased RBC turnover)
- Chronic renal failure
- Vitamin E supplementation
- Chronic blood loss

GLYCOSYLATED HEMOGLOBIN (A1C)

Increased with:
- Lead poisoning
- Thalassemia (RBC life span is longer)
- Acute stress response
- Cushing's syndrome
- Pheochromocytoma
- Glucagonoma
- Corticosteroid therapy
- Acromegaly
- Splenectomy

Medications that may increase levels:

Aspirin	Atenolol	Beta blockers
Gemfibrozil	Glimepiride	Hydrochlorothiazide
Indapamide	Lovastatin	Niacin
Nicardipine	Nicotinic acid	Propranolol

Medications that may decrease levels:

Acarbose	Deferoxamine	Diltiazem
Enalapril	Glipizide	Glyburide
Insulin	Lisinopril	Metformin
Nisoldipine	Pravastatin	Ramipril
Terazosin	Verapamil	

HEMATOCRIT (HCT) OR PACKED CELL VOLUME (PCV)

NORMAL VALUES
Newborn:	44-64%; 0.44-0.64 (SI)
2-8 wk:	39-59%; 0.39-0.59 (SI)
2-6 mos:	35-50%; 0.35-0.50 (SI)
6 mos-1 yr:	29-43%; 0.29-0.43 (SI)
1-6 y:	30-40%; 0.30-0.40 (SI)
6-18 yr:	32-44%; 0.32-0.44 (SI)
Adult females:	37-47%; 0.37-0.47 (SI)
Adult males:	42-52%; 0.42-0.52 (SI)

Values tend to be lower in the elderly

NUTRITIONAL SIGNIFICANCE

The word hematocrit means 'to separate blood.' Hematocrit is the measure of the percentage of RBC in total blood volume. Once the blood is centrifuged in a test tube, the height of the RBC column is compared to the height of the column of the total whole blood.

Hematocrit is a part of a routine CBC. It is used along with hemoglobin to evaluate iron status. Usually the hematocrit percentage is three times the hemoglobin concentration in grams per deciliter. This will not be the case if the RBC are of abnormal size or hemoglobin concentration is abnormal. Critical values are < 15 percent or > 60 percent.

The hematocrit value is affected by an extremely high WBC count and hydration status. It should be evaluated in light of other laboratory values. Individuals living in high altitudes often have increased values. It is common for individuals over the age of 50 to have slightly lower levels than younger adults. Individuals with inflammatory diseases will not be able to maintain normal

HEMATOCRIT (HCT) OR PACKED CELL VOLUME (PCV)

hematocrit levels because the body redistributes the iron from RBC to ferritin stores.

Normal hematocrit levels tend to be lower in individuals of African decent than for other ethnic groups. Individuals of Asian and Hispanic heritage tend to have higher levels than Caucasians.

Decisions concerning the need for a blood transfusion are often based on the hematocrit and hemoglobin. The older patient, with compromised oxygen-carrying capacity may benefit from a blood transfusion when the hematocrit reaches 30 percent. For younger patients, a transfusion is usually not considered until the hematocrit is < 24 percent.

RELATED TESTS: HGB, CBC, MCV, MCH, MCHC, RDW, serum iron, ferritin, TIBC

Increased with:
- Dehydration
- Shock
- Acute blood loss
- Erythrocytosis
- Polycythemia vera
- Surgery
- Burns
- High altitudes
- Severe diarrhea
- Eclampsia
- COPD
- Congenital heart disease

Decreased with:
- Overhydration
- Bone marrow failure
- Hyperthyroidism
- Hodgkin's disease
- Hemolytic anemia
- Prosthetic valves
- Renal disease
- Pregnancy
- Lymphoma
- Leukemia
- Adrenal insufficiency
- Multiple myeloma
- Hemolytic reaction
- Cirrhosis
- AIDS
- Hemorrhage
- Hemoglobinopathy

HEMATOCRIT (HCT) OR PACKED CELL VOLUME (PCV)

Decreased with:
- Rheumatoid arthritis
- Malnutrition/dietary deficiency

Medications that may increase levels:
Gentamicin Methyldopa

Medications that may decrease levels:
Antibiotics	Antineoplastic drugs	Aspirin
Chloramphenicol	Indomethacin	Penicillin
Rifampin	Sulfonamides	

HEMOGLOBIN (HGB)

NORMAL VALUES
Newborn:	12-14 g/dL; 7.5-8.7 mmol/L (SI)
2-8 wk:	12-20 g/dL; 7.5-12.4 mmol/L (SI)
2-6 mos:	10-17 g/dL; 6.2-10.6 mmol/L (SI)
6 mos-1 yr:	9.5-14 g/dL; 5.9- 8.7 mmol/L (SI)
1-6 yr:	9.5-14 g/dL; 5.9- 8.7 mmol/L (SI)
6-18 yr:	10-15.5 g/dL ; 6.2-9.6 mmol/L (SI)
Adult females:	12-16 g/dL; 7.4-9.9 mmol/L (SI)
Adult males:	14-18 g/dL; 8.7-11.2 mmol/L (SI)
Pregnant female:	> 11 g/dL ; 5.6mmol/L (SI)

Values tend to be lower in the elderly

NUTRITIONAL SIGNIFICANCE

Hemoglobin is the main component of RBC The hemoglobin concentration is a measure of the total amount of hemoglobin in the peripheral blood. It is a part of a routine CBC. It is a more direct measure of iron deficiency than hematocrit.

Hemoglobin is made up of heme and globin. The iron is surrounded by protoporphyrin. Abnormalities in the globin structure are called hemoglobinopathies. In these diseases the RBC count is low, the RBC survival rate and oxygen-carrying capacity are diminished.

Hemoglobin serves as a vehicle for oxygen and carbon dioxide transport. It picks up oxygen from the lungs and transports oxygen to the cells for oxidation reactions. From the cells, the hemoglobin carries carbon dioxide to the lungs to be exhaled. When the hemoglobin is low, the heart is strained to maintain good oxygen carrying capacity. When values hit critical levels (< 5 g/dL), the patient is at risk for angina, heart attack,

HEMOGLOBIN (HGB)

congestive heart failure and stroke. Decisions concerning the need for a blood transfusion are often based on the hematocrit and hemoglobin. The older patient, with compromised oxygen-carrying capacity may benefit from a blood transfusion when the hemoglobin reaches 8 g/dL. For younger patients, a transfusion is usually not considered until the hemoglobin is < 6 g/dL.

The normal hemoglobin is 1 g lower in individuals of African decent than for other ethnic groups. Individuals of Asian and Hispanic heritage tend to have higher levels than Caucasians. When hemoglobin levels are very high (> 20 g/dL), intravascular sludge occurs which increases the risk for stroke and other organ infarction. Changes in hydration status affect hemoglobin. Overhydration decreases the concentration and dehydration increases the concentration. Living in high altitudes may cause higher hemoglobin values.

Hemoglobin is involved with chloride in acid-base balance. The carbonic acid formed in RBC separates into H and HCO_3. The hydrogen ion binds to hemoglobin leaving the HCO_3 free to move out of the red blood cells. The electrical neutrality is maintained by chloride shifting into the RBC.

RELATED TESTS: HCT, CBC, MCV, MCH, MCHC, RDW, serum iron, ferritin, TIBC

Increased with:
- Dehydration
- High altitudes
- Polycythemia vera

Decreased with:
- Overhydration
- Iron deficiency anemia
- Pernicious anemia

HEMOGLOBIN (HGB)

Increased with:
- Severe burns
- Congestive heart failure
- Severe diarrhea
- Congenital heart disease
- Eclampsia
- COPD

Decreased with:
- Megaloblastic anemia
- Sickle cell anemia
- Hypertension
- Systemic diseases:
  - leukemia
  - lymphoma
  - erythematous
  - sarcoidosis
  - Hodgkin's disease
  - rheumatoid arthritis
  - systemic lupus
- Cirrhosis
- Hypothyroidism
- Cancer
- AIDS
- Multiple myeloma
- Splenomegaly
- Acute or chronic hemorrhage
- Neoplasia
- Thalassemia
- Hemolysis
- Hemoglobinopathies
- Malnutrition
- Prosthetic valves

Medications that may increase levels:
Gentamicin   Methyldopa

Medications that may decrease levels:
Antibiotics   Antineoplastic drugs   Aspirin
Chloramphenicol   Indomethacin   Penicillin
Rifampin   Sulfonamides

HOMOCYSTEINE (Hcy)

NORMAL VALUES
Adults: 0.54-2.3 mg/L; 4-14 µmol/L(SI)

NUTRITIONAL SIGNIFICANCE

Homocysteine is an intermediate metabolite of the methionine pathway. When methionine is released from dietary protein it condenses with adenosine triphosphate (ATP) to form S-adenosylmethionine (SAM). SAM acts as a methyl donor and homocysteine is formed. Homocysteine can either be remethylated to form methionine or catabolized in the transsulfuration pathway. The remethylation of homocysteine to methionine requires both vitamin B12 and folic acid. When vitamin B12 is deficient in the diet, the folic acid becomes trapped in an unusable form as methyltetrahydrofolate. A deficiency of folate acid results in megaloblastic anemia. Large doses of folic acid can override the pathway and mask a B12 deficiency.

Serum levels of homocysteine will rise when there is a B12 and/or a folic acid deficiency. The threshold for rising levels of homocysteine appears to be serum folate <12.5 nmol/L and/or serum B12 <225 pmol/L. Elevated levels are also associated with an increased risk for end stage renal disease, ischemic heart disease, cerebrovascular disease, peripheral arterial disease and venous thrombosis that are independent of lipid levels. While the etiology of the disease process is unclear, research suggests that elevated homocysteine levels promote the progression of atherosclerosis by causing endothelial damage, promoting LDL

HOMOCYSTEINE (Hcy)

deposition and promoting vascular smooth muscle growth. Individuals with progressive atherosclerosis despite normal lipoproteins should be screened for hyperhomocystinuria.

The most common etiology of an elevated homocysteine is a dietary deficiency of vitamins B6, B12 or folate. These vitamins are essential for the enzymatic metabolism of homocysteine to methionine. Some researchers have proposed that supplementation with vitamins B6, B12 and folate will reduce homocysteine levels and ultimately reduce risk of cardiovascular disease and renal disease. Reported data is inconclusive, however many studies are underway.

Elevated levels in pregnant women are associated with increased risk for neural tube defects and other complications.

Both fasting and post methionine loading levels of homocysteine can be measured. Patients whose creatinine levels are > 1.5 mg/dL are not candidates for methionine loading. The elevated creatinine levels suggest that the kidneys are unlikely to effectively filter the methionine.

Currently, homocysteine testing is not standardized and normal ranges vary. However, levels <12 µmol/L are optimal, levels 12-15 µmol/L are borderline and levels > 15 µmol/L are considered high risk for vascular disease. Men tend to have higher homocysteine levels than women, possibly due to higher creatinine values and greater muscle mass. Smoking is associated with higher levels of homocysteine.

HOMOCYSTEINE (Hcy)

RELATED TESTS: serum B6, serum B12, lipoproteins, cholesterol, triglyceride, apolipoproteins

Increased with:
- Renal failure
- Folate deficiency
- B12 deficiency
- B6 deficiency
- Malnutrition
- Cardiovascular disease
- Homocystinuria
- Cerebrovascular disease
- Peripheral vascular disease
- Cystinuria
- Osteoporosis

Medications that may increase levels:

Azaribine	Carbamazepine	Methotrexate
Nitrous oxide	Theophylline	Phenytoin

Mediations that may decrease levels:

Folic acid	Penicillamine
Oral contraceptives	Tamoxifen

Iron Level (Serum Fe, Total Iron Binding Capacity (TIBC), Transferrin, Transferrin Saturation)

Normal Values
Serum Fe
  Females: 60-160 mcg/dL; 11-29 μmol/L (SI)
  Males: 80-180 mcg/dL; 14-32 μmol/L (SI)

TIBC   250-460 mcg/dL; 45-82 μmol/L (SI)

Transferrin
  Females: 250-380 mg/dL; 2.50-3.80 g/L (SI)
  Males: 215-365 mg/dL; 2.15-3.65 g/L (SI)

Transferrin Saturation
  Females: 15%-50%
  Males: 20%-50%

Nutritional Significance

Seventy percent of the iron in the body is found in the hemoglobin of the RBC. Dietary iron is absorbed in the small intestine and transported to the plasma where it is bound to transferrin and transported to the bone marrow for production of hemoglobin. The remaining 30 percent of iron is stored as ferritin and hemosiderin in the liver and other tissues for future use. Iron is bound to a globulin protein called transferrin. The serum iron reflects the amount of iron bound to transferrin.

Serum iron is reduced in iron deficiency anemia. Iron deficiency may be caused by insufficient intake, poor gut absorption, increased needs or increased losses. In all cases, there is a decreased production of hemoglobin. The RBC become smaller and paler in color. Iron deficiency anemia is a microcytic hypochromic anemia. Diagnostic values include low hemoglobin,

Iron Level (Serum Fe, Total Iron Binding Capacity (TIBC), Transferrin, Transferrin Saturation)

hematocrit, serum iron, transferrin saturation and elevated TIBC.

During inflammatory stress, cytokines impair the production of erythrocytes and reorient iron stores from hemoglobin and serum iron to ferritin. During infection IL-1β inhibits the production and release of transferrin while stimulating the synthesis of ferritin. Laboratory test results used to predict the risk of nutritional anemias are not useful in assessing the patient with inflammatory response. As inflammatory process wanes, the iron stores will shift from ferritin to hemoglobin and transferrin.

Hemochromatosis or hemosiderosis is iron overload or poisoning. Excess iron is stored in the brain, liver and heart resulting in severe dysfunction. Massive blood transfusions may contribute to iron overload. Metabolic disorders atransferrinemia, porphyria and cutanea tarda are characterized with iron overload.

TIBC is a direct measure of all proteins available to bind mobile iron. Transferrin represents the largest quantity of iron-binding proteins. TIBC is an indirect measurement of transferrin stores except in cases of iron overload. Transferrin levels are normal or decreased with iron overload. Other, less common iron-carrying proteins, increase in number during iron overload. Ferritin is not included in TICB because it only binds with stored iron. TIBC is elevated in about 70 percent of patients of iron deficiency anemia.

Iron Level (Serum Fe, Total Iron Binding Capacity (TIBC), Transferrin, Transferrin Saturation)

When TIBC is not available, transferrin can be directly measured. The percentage of saturation of transferrin can be calculated by dividing the serum iron level by the TIBC. This calculation is helpful in determining the cause of abnormal iron and TIBC levels. Transferrin saturation is decreased to < 15 percent with iron deficiency anemia. It is increased in patients with iron overload or iron poisoning, hemolytic, sideroblastic and megaloblastic anemias. Increased intake or absorption seen in hemochromatosis leads to elevated iron levels. The TICB is normal, but the transferrin saturation is very high.

Transferrin is also a negative acute phase reactant protein. Levels diminish when acute inflammatory reactions occur. Transferrin is also lower in patients with malignancies, collagen vascular diseases and liver diseases. Serum iron and TIBC will be depressed, but transferrin saturation will be normal. Hypoproteinemia is also associated with reduced transferrin levels.

Related Tests: ferritin, RBC indices

Serum Fe Increased with:
- Pernicious anemia
- Aplastic anemia
- Hemolytic anemia
- B_6 deficiency
- Thalassemia
- Acute hepatitis
- Repeated transfusions
- Nephritis
- Excessive iron therapy

Serum Fe Decreased with:
- Iron deficiency anemia
- Acute and chronic infection
- Cancer
- Malnutrition
- Nephrosis
- Insufficient dietary iron
- Diverticulosis
- Inadequate iron absorption
- Pregnancy

Iron Level (Serum Fe, Total Iron Binding Capacity (TIBC), Transferrin, Transferrin Saturation)

Serum Fe Increased with:
- Hemosiderosis
- Hemochromatosis
- Hepatic necrosis
- Lead poisoning
- Massive transfusions
- Iron poisoning
- Acute leukemia

Serum Fe Decreased with:
- Chronic blood loss
- Chronic hematuria
- Chronic heavy menstruation
- Chronic GI blood loss
- Inflammatory bowel disease

Medications that may increase Serum Fe levels:

Acetylsalicylic acid	Cefotaxime	Chemotherapeutic agents
Chloramphenicol	Cisplatin	Dextran
Estrogen	Ethanol	Methicillin
Methimazole	Methotrexate	Methyldopa
Multivitamins	Oral contraceptives	Pyrazinamide

Medications that may decrease Serum Fe levels:

ACTH	Allopurinol	Aspirin
Cholestyramine	Colchicine	Corticotropin
Cortisone	Deferoxamine	Metformin
Methicillin	Oxymetholone	Pergolide
Risperidone	Testosterone	

Transferrin Increased with:
- Dehydration
- Iron deficiency anemia
- Pregnancy (3rd Trimester)
- Hepatitis
- Chronic blood loss
- Polycythemia vera

Transferrin Decreased with:
- Overhydration
- Pernicious anemia
- Chronic infection
- Liver disease
- Acute catabolic stress
- Malnutrition
- Nephrotic syndrome
- Iron overload
- Sickle cell anemia
- Burns
- Anemia of chronic & inflammatory diseases
- AIDS

Iron Level (Serum Fe, Total Iron Binding Capacity (TIBC), Transferrin, Transferrin Saturation)

TIBC Increased with:
- Iron deficiency anemia
- Polycythemia vera
- Pregnancy
- Acute hepatitis
- Acute and chronic blood loss

TIBC Decreased with:
- Hypoproteinemia
- Inflammatory diseases
- Cirrhosis
- Hemolytic anemia
- Pernicious anemia
- Thalassemia
- Malnutrition
- Hyperthyroidism
- Sickle cell anemia

Medications that may increase TIBC or Transferrin:
Fluorides   Oral contraceptives

Medications that may decrease TIBC or Transferrin:
ACTH   Chloramphenicol

Transferrin Saturation Increased with:
- Hemochromatosis
- Hemosiderosis
- ↑ Fe intake
- Hemolytic anemia
- Acute liver disease
- Thalassemia

Transferrin Saturation Decreased with:
- Iron deficiency anemia
- Chronic illness
- Malignancy
- Anemia of chronic & inflammatory diseases

LACTIC DEHYDROGENASE (LDH)

NORMAL VALUES
Newborn:	160-450 U/L; 160-450 U/L(SI)
Infant:	100-250 U/L; 100-250 U/L(SI)
Child:	60-170 U/L; 60-170 U/L (SI)
Adult/Elderly:	100 - 190 U/L at 37° C; 100 - 190 U/L (SI)

Isoenzymes in adult/elderly:
LDH-1:	17% - 27%; 0.17-0.27 of total
LDH-2:	27% - 37%; 0.27-0.37 of total
LDH-3:	18% - 25%; 0.18- 0.25 of total
LDH-4:	3% - 8%; 0.03-0.08 of total
LDH-5:	0% - 5%; 0.0 -0.05 of total

NUTRITIONAL SIGNIFICANCE

Lactic dehydrogenase (LDH) is an enzyme found in heart, liver, skeletal muscle, brain, red blood cells and lung cells. LDH is not a specific indicator of any one disease affecting one organ. When disease or injury affects cells, the cells lyse and release LDH.

Five isoenzymes of lactic dehydrogenase can be separated by electrophoresis. LDH-1 comes mainly from heart and blood vessels; LDH-2 primarily from the reticuloendothelial system; LDH-3 comes from the lungs; LDH-4 comes from the kidney, placenta and pancreas; LDH-5 comes from the liver and striated muscle.

LDH-2 levels are normally higher than the other isoenzymes. When LDH-1 is elevated above LDH-2 (LDH flip), it suggests a possible hemolytic anemia, megaloblastic anemia and/or sickle cell anemia. The time elapsed to peak values is used to differentiate these conditions. The LDH flipped ratio is also

Lactic Dehydrogenase (LDH)

seen in a myocardial infarction. However newer cardiac markers have replaced LDH as a diagnostic criterion for myocardial infarction.

An isolated elevation of LHD-5 suggests hepatocellular injury or disease. Elevation of LDH-2 and LDH-3 indicates pulmonary injury or disease. If all the LDH isoenzymes are elevated, this indicates multi-organ failure or advanced malignancy or diffuse autoimmune inflammatory disease. In patients with multiple co-morbidities, more than one disease may be causing an elevation in different LDH isoenzymes making the lab results inconclusive. LDH is also measured in the urine. Elevated levels indicate neoplasm or injury to the urologic system.

Related Tests: AST, GGTP, ALP, 5-nucleotidase, CK, ALT, LAP

Increased with:
- Myocardial infarction
- CNS diseases
- Pulmonary disease:
    - pneumonia
    - pulmonary embolism
    - pulmonary infarction
- Hepatic diseases:
    - hepatitis
    - cirrhosis
    - neoplasm
    - alcoholism
- Skeletal muscle disease & injury:
    - muscular dystrophy
    - muscular trauma
- Heat stroke

Decreased with:
- Good response to cancer therapy

LACTIC DEHYDROGENASE (LDH)

Increased with:
- Pancreatitis
- Red blood cell diseases:
  - RBC lyse due to prosthetic heart valves
- Anemias
  - sickle cell
  - megaloblastic
  - pernicious anemia
  - hemolytic anemia
- Shock
- Renal parenchymal diseases
  - infarction
  - glomerulonephritis
  - acute tubular necrosis
  - uremia
  - kidney transplant rejection
- Cancers
  - lymphoma, testicular, leukemia
- Intestinal ischemia and infarction
- Cerebrovascular accident
- Infectious mononucleosis
- Fracture
- Hypotension
- Congestive heart failure
- Hypoxia
- Delirium tremens
- Seizures
- Hyperthermia
- Hypothyroidism
- Hypoxia
- Head injury
- Intestinal obstruction

Medications that may increase levels:
Acebutolol	Alcohol	Amiodarone
Amphotericin B	Anabolic steroids	Anesthetic agents

Lactic Dehydrogenase (LDH)

Medications that may increase levels:

Aripiprazole	Aspirin	Auranofin
Azithromycin	Betaxolol	Captopril
Carbenicillin	Cefdinir	Cefonicid
Cefotaxime	Cefotetan	Cefoxitin
Cefpodoxime	Ceftazidime	Cefuroxime
Chloramphenicol	Chlordane	Chlorpromazine
Chlorpropamide	Chlortetracycline	Chlorthalidone
Cimetidine	Ciprofloxacin	Clindamycin
Clofibrate	Codeine	Dapsone
Diclofenac	Diltiazem	Donepezil
Doxorubicin	Estramustine	Etretinate
Fenoprofen	Floxuridine	Fluorides
Fluphenazine	Fluvoxamine	Foscarnet
Furosemide	Ganciclovir	Gentamicin
Gold	Granulocyte colonizing factor	Hydralazine
Ibuprofen	Imipramine	Interferon-alfa-2a
Interleukin-2	Isotretinoin	Itraconazole
Levodopa	Meperidine	Mesalamine
Methotrexate	Methyldopa	Metoprolol
Mithramycin	Morphine	Mycophenolate
Nefazodone	Nelfinavir	Nifedipine
Nitrofurantoin	Norfloxacin	Ofloxacin
Oxacillin	Oxaprozin	Paroxetine
Pegfilgrastim	Pemoline	Penicillamine
Pindolol	Piperacillin	Plicamycin
Procainamide	Propoxyphene	Propranolol
Propylthiouracil	Quinidine	Quinupristin/dalfopristin
Riluzole	Sibutramine	Simvastatin
Streptokinase	Streptozocin	Sulfamethoxazole
Sulfasalazine	Sulfisoxazole	Sulindac
Tobramycin	Tolmetin	Valproic acid
Vasopressin	Verapamil	

Medications that may decrease levels:

Amikacin	Anticonvulsants	Ascorbic acid
Cefotaxime	Clofibrate	Enalapril
Hydroxyurea	Metronidazole	Naltrexone

MAGNESIUM (Mg^{++}), SERUM & URINE

NORMAL VALUES, SERUM
Newborn:	1.5-2.2 mEq/L; 0.62-0.91 mmol/L (SI)
Child:	1.7-2.1 mEq/L; 0.70-0.86 mmol/L (SI)
Adult:	1.8-2.6 mEq/L; 0.74-1.07 mmol/L (SI)

CRITICAL VALUES
Hypomagnesemia:	< 1.2 mg/dL; < 0.49 mmol/L (SI)
Hypermagnesemia:	> 5.0 mg/dL; > 2.1 mmol/L (SI)

NUTRITIONAL SIGNIFICANCE

Magnesium is the second most abundant cation (after potassium) in the body. It is found in the bone (40-60 percent), muscle (20 percent), within cells (30 percent) and serum (1 percent). About half of the magnesium found in blood is free, 1/3 is bound to albumin and the balance is complexed with citrate, phosphate or other anions.

Magnesium is required for the use of ATP for energy and is involved in carbohydrate metabolism, protein synthesis, nucleic acid synthesis and contraction of muscles. In conjunction with sodium, potassium and calcium ions, it also regulates neuromuscular irritability and blood clotting. It is difficult to maintain normal potassium levels when magnesium is low.

Magnesium and calcium are intimately linked. A deficiency of either has significant effect on the metabolism of the other. Magnesium is involved in the absorption of calcium from the intestines and in calcium metabolism. A deficiency of magnesium will result in a drift of calcium out of the bones into soft tissues, including the aorta and kidneys.

Magnesium (Mg^{++}), Serum & Urine

In healthy adults, 95 percent of the magnesium is filtered through the glomerulus and reabsorbed in the tubule. With compromised kidney function, greater amounts of magnesium are retained, resulting in increased serum levels.

Magnesium deficiency may occur in individuals who are malnourished. Deficiency symptoms include weakness, irritability, tetany, electrocardiographic changes, delirium and convulsions. In magnesium deficiency, urinary magnesium declines before the serum levels. Serum magnesium levels may remain within normal ranges even when total body stores are depletes up to 20 percent. Magnesium deficiency is also related to hypocalcemia and hypokalemia. Common neurologic and GI symptoms associated with these cases include muscle tremors, muscle twitching and tetany, anorexia, nausea, vomiting, ECG abnormalities, insomnia, delirium, convulsions and hyperactive deep tendon reflexes.

Increased magnesium levels may be due to ingestion of magnesium containing antacids and exacerbated by chronic renal insufficiency or chronic renal failure. Symptoms of elevated magnesium levels include lethargy, nausea, vomiting, flushing, weak or absent deep tendon reflexes, hypotension, drowsiness, respiratory depression, slurred speech and ECG abnormalities. Specific symptoms associated with various level of hypermagnesemia are noted in Table 22.

Magnesium (Mg++), Serum & Urine

Table 22. Symptoms Associated with Hypermagnesemia

Magnesium Level (serum)	Symptoms
5.0-10.0 mg/dL: 2.1-4.1 mmol/L	CNS depression, nausea, vomiting, fatigue
10-15 mg/dL ; 4.1-6.2 mmol/L	Coma, ECG changes, respiratory paralysis
30 mg/dL ; 12.3 mmol/L	Complete heart block
34-40 mg/dL ; 14-16 mmol/L	Cardiac arrest

Related Tests: kidney function tests, potassium, sodium, calcium

Serum Mg++ Increased with:
- Renal insufficiency & failure
- Uncontrolled diabetes
- Addison's' disease
- Hypothyroidism
- Dehydration
- Antacids containing Mg++
- Oliguria

Serum Mg++ Decreased with:
- Malnutrition
- Malabsorption
- Hypoparathyroidism
- Alcoholism
- Chronic renal disease
- Diabetic acidosis
- Hypercalcemia
- Chronic pancreatitis
- Hyperaldosteronism
- Long term TPN
- SIADH
- Pregnancy (2nd, 3rd trimester)
- Excessive loss of body fluids
  - diaphoresis
  - lactation
  - diuretic abuse
  - chronic diarrhea

Magnesium (Mg++), Serum & Urine

Medications that may increase serum levels:
Alkaline antacids	Amiloride	Aminoglycoside antibiotics
Antacids	Aspirin	Calcitriol
Cefotaxime	Felodipine	Hydroflumethiazide
Lithium	Loop diuretics	Magnesium salts
Medroxyprogesterone	Progesterone	Sodium bicarbonate
Tacrolimus	Thyroid medications	Triamterene

Medications that may decrease serum levels:
Albuterol	Aldesleukin	Amphotericin B
Arsenic trioxide	Azathioprine	Basiliximab
Calcitriol	Calcium gluconate	Cefotaxime
Chlorothiazide	Chlorthalidone	Cisplatin
Cyclosporine	Digoxin	Doxorubicin
Ethacrynic acid	Foscarnet	Furosemide
Gentamicin	Haloperidol	Hydrochlorothiazide
Hydroflumethiazide	Insulin	Metolazone
Neomycin	Oral contraceptives	Pamidronate
Pentamidine	Prednisolone	Sirolimus
Tacrolimus	Theophylline	Thiazides
Tobramycin	Trastuzumab	Voriconazole
Zalcitabine	Zoledronic acid	

Medications that may increase urine levels:
Acetazolamide	Ammonia chloride	Amphotericin B
Bumetanide	Calcitonin	Chlorothiazide
Cisplatin	Cyclosporin A	Ethacrynic
Furosemide	Gentamicin	Hydrochlorothiazide
Lithium	Magnesium hydroxide	Methyclothiazide
Thiazides	Torsemide	Triamterene

Medications that may decrease urine levels:
Acetazolamide	Amiloride	Calcium gluconate
Interferon α-2a	Oral contraceptives	Parathyroid extract

Methyl Malonic Acid (MMA), Serum & Urine

Normal Values
Adults: Serum   17-76 ng/mL; 0.08 to 0.56 µmol/L (SI)
Adults: Urine   <5 mg/day

Nutritional Significance

Methyl malonic acid (MMA) is an intermediate metabolite of catabolism of certain amino acids, odd chain fatty acids and other compounds that produce propionyl coenzyme A (CoA). The end result of these metabolic pathways is succinyl CoA that enters the Kreb cycle. The normal pathway requires cobalamin (B12) to convert L-methylmalonyl CoA to succinyl CoA. When vitamin B12 is deficient, an excess of D-methylmalonyl CoA is hydrolyzed to MMA.

This test is a sensitive and early indicator of declining tissue levels of vitamin B12. Increased serum concentrations of MMA are often detectible before hematologic changes are noted. Some patients with elevated levels of MMA may not have any symptoms while others may report neurological changes including numbness and tingling in the hands and feet or cognitive or behavioral changes such as confusion, irritability or depression.

Urinary MMA is measured using a random urine sample. The value is normalized to urine creatine to correct for urine dilution. The urinary MMA/creatinine ratio (uMMA test) is more accurate than the serum MMA because it indicates tissue level vitamin B12 deficiency.

Methyl Malonic Acid (MMA), Serum & Urine

MMA testing is useful to differentiate between a vitamin B12 and folate deficiency. Levels are elevated in pernicious anemia but normal in folate deficiency. Levels may be elevated in chronic renal failure because of a decreased excretion of MMA in the urine.

An elevated MMA level does not necessarily reflect the severity of the vitamin B12 deficiency. Some studies have reported a considerable variation of MMA levels over time.

Related Tests: homocysteine, serum B12.

Increased with:
- Pernicious anemia
- Chronic renal failure

NATRIURETIC PEPTIDES (ATRIAL NATRIURETIC PEPTIDE, BRAIN NATRIURETIC PEPTIDE, N-TERMINAL FRAGMENT OF PRO-BRAIN NATRIURETIC PEPTIDE)

NORMAL VALUES

Atrial Natriuretic Peptide (ANP):   22-77 pg/mL; 22-77 ng/L (SI)
Brain Natriuretic Peptide (BNP):   < 100 pg/mL; < 100 ng/L(SI)

N-terminal fragment of Pro-Brain Natriuretic Peptide: (NT-pro-BNP): Healthy males: < or = to 60 pg/mL; < or = to 60 ng/L (SI)
Healthy females: 12-125 pg/mL; 12-125 ng/L (SI)
Elderly: levels increase with age

NT-pro-BNP for Acute Heart Failure:
Adults <50 yr: 450 pg/mL; 450 ng/L(SI)
Adults 50–75 yr: 900 pg/mL; 900 ng/L(SI)
Adults >75 yr: 1800 pg/mL; 1800 ng/L(SI)

NUTRITIONAL SIGNIFICANCE

Natriuretic peptides are a group of substances that counter the activity of the renin-angiotensin system. The Atrial Natriuretic Peptide (ANP) is synthesized in the cardiac atrial muscle. The Brain Natriuretic Peptide (BNP) is synthesized in the cardiac ventricular muscle. Both ANP and BNP are released in response to atrial and ventricular stretch and will cause vasorelaxation and block secretion of aldosterone from the adrenal gland and renin from the kidney. The end result is an increased glomerular filtration rate, decreased sodium retention urinary excretion and a reduction in blood volume. The higher the level of BNP, the more severe is the congestive heart failure (CHF). In some labs the BNP is measured as an N-terminal fragment of Pro-Brain Natriuretic Peptide (NT-pro-BNP), a precursor form of BNP. The NT-pro-

NATRIURETIC PEPTIDES (ATRIAL NATRIURETIC PEPTIDE, BRAIN NATRIURETIC PEPTIDE, N-TERMINAL FRAGMENT OF PRO-BRAIN NATRIURETIC PEPTIDE)

BNP is a stronger predictor of mortality among patients with acute and chronic coronary syndromes.

BNP and NT-pro-BNP increase in response to ventricular volume expansion and pressure overload, thus serving as good markers for cardiac dysfunction. NT-pro-BNP values above 125 pg/mL; 125 ng/L may indicate the presence of early cardiac dysfunction and are associated with increased risk of myocardial infarction, heart failure or death. NT-pro-BNP is used for CHF risk stratification. CHF patients whose NT-pro-BNP levels does not rapidly return to normal with treatment experience a significantly higher risk of mortality than those whose levels rapidly normalize. NT-pro-BNP is elevated in early rejection of heart transplants and in those with prolonged systemic hypertension. Results for BNP and NT-pro-BNP are not interchangeable and can not be compared.

RELATED TESTS: blood pressure

Increased with:
- Diastolic dysfunction
- Congestive heart failure
- Myocardial infarction
- Systemic hypertension
- Heart transplant rejection

Natriuretic Peptides (Atrial Natriuretic Peptide, Brain Natriuretic Peptide, N-terminal Fragment of Pro-Brain Natriuretic Peptide)

Medications that may cause increased ANP levels:

Atenolol	Captopril	Carteolol
Cyclosporine	Dipyridamole	Doxorubicin
Morphine	Nifedipine	Oral contraceptives
Vasopressin	Verapamil	

Medications that may cause decreased ANP levels:

Benazepril	Chlorthalidone	Clonidine
Erythropoietin	Methimazole	Prazosin
Ramipril		

OSMOLALITY, SERUM

NORMAL VALUES
Newborns: as low as 266 mOsm/kg H2O; 266 mmol/kg H2O (SI)
Child: 275 – 290 mOsm/kg H2O; 275-290 mmol/kg H2O (SI)
Adult/elderly: 285 - 295 mOsm/kg H2O; 285-295 mmol/kg H2O (SI)

OSMOLAL GAP
Adults: 5-10 mOsm/kg H2O; 5-10 mmol/kg H_2O (SI)

NUTRITIONAL SIGNIFICANCE

Osmolality measures the concentration of dissolved particles in a solution. When free water in the blood increases or the number of particles decreases, osmolality decreases. This is overhydration. Critical values for overhydration are less than 265 mOsm/kg H2O.

When the amount of water in the blood decreases or the number of particles increases, osmolality increases. This is dehydration. Critical values for dehydration are > 320 mOsm/kg H2O. When serum osmolality increases the antidiuretic hormone is secreted causing more water reabsorption, more concentrated urine and a less concentrated serum. When serum osmolality is low the body decreases water reabsorption and excretes large amounts of dilute urine.

Serum osmolality is used to evaluate fluid and electrolyte imbalance, seizures, ascites, liver disease, hydration status, acid-base balance and ADH abnormalities. Osmolality is also used to identify ethanol, sugars or ketones in the blood. When present in abnormal amounts there is an 'osmolal gap.'

OSMOLALITY, SERUM

The gap refers to the difference between the actual and calculated osmolality. The gap is usually due to the presence of ketones, glucose or ethanol by-products. Hypertriglyceridemia and hyperproteinemia can cause an elevated osmolal gap. An osmolal gap of > 10 mOsm/kg H2O is seen in severely ill patients, those in shock, with lactic acidosis and in renal failure.
Serum osmolality is used to evaluate patients in coma. Critical values are those > 320 mOsm/kg H2O. However, > 385 mOsm/kg H2O are associated with stupor in patients with hyperglycemia. Levels between 400-420 mOsm/kg/H2O; 400-420 mmol/kg H2O are associated with grand mal seizures. Death can occur when levels are > 420 mOsm/kg H2O.

RELATED TESTS: urine osmolality, ADH, ADH suppression test

Increased with:
- Hypernatremia
- Dehydration
- Hyperglycemia
- Azotemia
- Shock
- Ingestion of ethanol, glycol, methanol, or ethylene
- Uremia
- Hyperosmolar nonketotic hyperglycemia
- Diabetes insipidus
- Hypercalcemia
- Renal tubular necrosis
- Severe pyelonephritis
- Ketosis
- Cerebral lesions

Decreased with:
- Hyponatremia
- Overhydration
- SIADH
- Panhypopituitarism
- Ascites
- Suspected ADH abnormalities
- Adrenocortical insufficiency
- Excessive water replacement
- Renal failure
- Paraneoplastic syndromes

OSMOLALITY, URINE

NORMAL FINDINGS
24 hr: 300-900 mOsm/kg H2O; 300-900 mmol/kg H2O (SI)
After 12 hr fluid restriction: >850 mOsm/kg H2O; >850 mmol/kg H2O
Random specimen: 50-1400 mOsm/kg H2O; 50-1400 mmol/kg H2O
Ratio of urine/serum osmolality: 0.2-4.7

NUTRITIONAL SIGNIFICANCE
    Urine osmolality is a measure of the number of dissolved particles in a solution. It is a more exact measurement of urine concentration than specific gravity. Specific gravity varies based on the number and type of particles in the urine.

    The urine of patients with glucosuria or proteinuria will have an 'osmolal gap' because of the presence of organic osmolar particles. Normally the osmolal gap is 80-100 mOsm/kg of H2O. The urine osmolality test results are more easily interpreted when the serum osmolality is simultaneously performed. The normal ratio between urine and serum osmolality is 1:3.

    Urine osmolality is used to evaluate the ability of the kidney to concentrate urine, to evaluate for acute and chronic renal failure, monitor electrolyte and water balance and to evaluate hydration status. It is also used to investigate ADH abnormalities as seen in diabetes insipidus and inappropriate ADH secretion. When ADH secretions are inadequate, the kidney's ability to concentrate urine is diminished and urine osmolality decreases.

OSMOLALITY, URINE

Urine osmolality will increase in certain medical conditions in which the kidneys reabsorb large quantities of free body water. Patients with congestive heart failure and other illnesses associated with edema due to reduced perfusion of the kidneys will have increased urine osmolality because less free body water is excreted. Patients in shock also experience a rise in urine osmolality. The normal physiological response to shock is to minimize loss of free body water. The kidneys will reabsorb all free body water and urine osmolality will increase.

RELATED TESTS: serum osmolality, ADH, ADH suppression

Increased with:
- SIADH
- Acidosis
- Shock
- Hypernatremia
- Hepatic cirrhosis
- Congestive heart disease
- Addison's disease
- Paraneoplastic syndromes (cancer of lung, breast, colon)
- Dehydration
- Amyloidosis

Decreased with:
- Diabetes insipidus
- Hypercalcemia
- Excess fluid intake
- Renal tubular necrosis
- Aldosteronism
- Hypokalemia
- Severe pyelonephritis

Phosphate (PO4, Phosphorus)

Normal Values
Newborn:	4.5-9.0 mg/dL; 1.45-2.91 mmol/L (SI)
Child:	4.5-5.5 mg/dL; 1.45-1.78 mmol/L (SI)
Adult:	2.7-4.5 mg/dL; 0.87-1.45 mmol/L (SI)

Nutritional Significance

The majority of phosphate found in the body is part of other organic compounds. Inorganic forms include phosphorus combined with calcium in the skeleton and the phosphate salt found in blood. Dietary phosphorus is absorbed in the small bowel. Hypophosphatemia is rare, but can be due to malabsorption and refeeding syndrome. Symptoms include tingling paresthesias in the tongue, fingers, and toes but can progress to severe weakness and areflexia, sensory loss, and cranial neuropathies. Neurologic manifestations can include ataxia, myoclonus, myopathy, myelopathy, dementia, and a peripheral neuropathy that can include sensorimotor axonal neuropathy, axonal motor and mononeuropathy multiplex.

Critical values are < 1 mg/dL; < 0.32 mmol/L.

Phosphate is required for the synthesis of bony tissue and functions in the metabolism of lipids and glucose. It is vital for acid-base balance and in the storage and transfer of energy from one site in the body to another. after consumption or infusion of carbohydrate.

Serum phosphorus levels are determined by calcium metabolism, parathyroid hormone (PTH), renal excretion and intestinal absorption. There is an inverse relationship between

Phosphate (PO4, Phosphorus)

calcium and phosphorus. A decrease in one mineral results in an increase in the other. Recent ingestion of carbohydrate including IV glucose, can cause a decrease in serum levels because phosphorus enters the cell with glucose.

    Refeeding syndrome occurs when previously malnourished patients are fed with high carbohydrate loads via tubefeeding or TPN. The delivery of glucose, either enterally or parenterally, can cause a huge increase in the circulating insulin level. There is rapid uptake of glucose, potassium, phosphate and magnesium into cells. The result is a rapid fall in serum phosphate, magnesium and potassium, along with an increasing ECF volume. Feeding slowly and aggressively supplementing with magnesium, phosphate and potassium is helpful to prevent refeeding syndrome.

    Disease states also influence the levels of phosphorous in the blood. In hyperparathyroidism, renal reabsorption is enhanced. In hyperparathyroidism, the PTH increases urinary excretion of phosphates. In kidney failure, phosphorus excretion diminishes significantly and serum levels rise.

    Phosphate is part of the body's buffering system. In acidosis, the pH is reduced, and phosphates are driven out of the cell and into the blood stream. In alkalosis, the pH is increasing and phosphate levels shift into cells causing hypophosphatemia.

Related Tests: PTH, serum calcium

Phosphate (PO4, Phosphorus)

Increased Levels with:
- Renal failure
- Increased dietary intake
- Acromegaly
- Hypothyroidism
- Bone metastasis
- Sarcoidosis
- Hypocalcemia
- Liver failure
- Acidosis
- Excessive intake vitamin D
- Milk-alkali syndrome
- Addison's disease
- Rhabdomyolysis
- Hypoparathyroidism
- Hemolytic anemia
- Advanced lymphoma or myeloma
- Healing fractures
- Cardiac resuscitation

Decreased Levels with:
- Inadequate dietary intake
- Chronic antacid ingestion
- Hyperparathyroidism
- Hypercalcemia
- Chronic alcoholism
- Vitamin D deficiency
- DKA
- Hyperinsulinism
- Osteomalacia
- Malnutrition
- Refeeding syndrome
- Respiratory alkalosis
- Sepsis
- Ricketts
- Vomiting
- Severe diarrhea
- Prolonged hypothermia

Medications that may cause increased levels:

Aldesleukin	Aluminium hydroxide	Anabolic steroids
Aspirin	Azithromycin	Basiliximab
Bisoprolol	Cefdinir	Cefotaxime
Dipyridamole	Epoetin alfa	Erythropoietin
Estramustine	Etidronate	Etretinate
Foscarnet	Furosemide	Growth hormone
Hydrochlorothiazide	Mannitol	Medroxyprogesterone
Methicillin	Methotrexate	Methyltestosterone
Minocycline	Nafarelin	Naproxen
Nifedipine	Nitrofurantoin	Oral contraceptives
Paroxetine	Phospho-soda	Pindolol
Rifampin	Risedronate	Risperidone
Sirolimus	Tacrolimus	Tetracycline
Theophylline	Timolol	Venlafaxine
Vitamin D		

PHOSPHATE (PO4, PHOSPHORUS)

Medications that may cause decreased levels:

Acetazolamide	Albuterol	Aldesleukin
Alendronate	Alkaline antacids	Aluminium salts
Amino acids	Amlodipine	Anesthetic agents
Anticonvulsants	Azathioprine	Calcitonin
Calcitriol	Carbamazepine	Cefdinir
Cisplatin	Doxorubicin	Etretinate
Foscarnet	Hydrochlorothiazide	Insulin
Isoniazid	Lithium	Mannitol
Mestranol	Mycophenolate	Niacin
Nicardipine	Oral contraceptives	Pamidronate
Phenothiazine	Phenytoin	Plicamycin
Raloxifene	Sirolimus	Sucralfate
Tacrolimus	Theophylline	Venlafaxine
Zoledronic acid		

POTASSIUM (K$^+$), SERUM

NORMAL VALUES
Neonates (0-7 days):	3.7 - 5.9 mEq/L; 3.7 - 5.9 mmol/L (SI)
Infants :	4.1 - 5.3 mEq/L; 4.1 - 5.3 mmol/L (SI)
Child:	3.4 – 4.7 mEq/L; 3.4 – 4.7 mmol/L (SI)
Adults:	3.5 - 5.2 mEq/L; 3.5 - 5.2 mmol/L (SI)

NUTRITIONAL SIGNIFICANCE

Potassium is the principle intracellular cation. The normal potassium level within cells is approximately 150 mEq/L compared to 3.5 - 5.0 mEq/L in serum. The level of potassium found outside the cells is the level measured by this laboratory test. The ratio of intracellular to extracellular potassium is of crucial importance in maintaining membrane electrical charges.

As a positively charged ion, potassium is involved in regulating the osmolarity of the extracellular fluid by exchanging with sodium. Its level is essential to maintain the transmembrane electrical potential between the intracellular fluid and the extracellular fluid.

The role of potassium is interrelated with the role of sodium. Both ions are involved with active transport processes. When sodium ions are pumped into the cell, potassium ions are pumped out of the cell. The sodium-potassium pump plays a key role in maintaining normal neuromuscular contractions. Even small changes in potassium concentrations can have significant consequences.

The serum potassium concentration is related to renin-aldosterone mechanism, sodium reabsorption and acid-base

Potassium (K⁺), Serum

balance. The renin-aldosterone mechanism is mediated by angiotensin. This mechanism stimulates the secretion of aldosterone to the distal tubule and affects potassium levels. Aldosterone stimulates an increased reabsorption of sodium. This action forces potassium to move in the opposite direction. In other words, potassium moves from the serum into the tubule for excretion. Aldosterone also stimulates potassium uptake in the proximal tubule. This process results in passive diffusion of potassium into the tubular lumen for excretion at the distal tubule. The body's ability to regulate sodium levels impacts potassium levels too. When an increased amount of sodium enters the distal tubule, the rate of sodium reabsorption by the distal end of the tubules and collecting ducts increases proportionately. Because potassium normally moves in the opposite direction of sodium, the potassium excretion increases and serum levels drop.

Potassium plays a vital role in nerve conduction, muscle function and osmotic pressure. Along with calcium and magnesium, potassium controls the rate and force of contraction of the heart (i.e. cardiac output). Evidence of a potassium deficit can be noted on ECG by the presence of a U wave.

Medical conditions that contribute to natriuresis result in a significant loss of potassium and an increased osmotic load due to the overhydration. The larger the osmotic load delivered to the proximal tubule the less potassium is reabsorbed. In other words, more potassium is lost via the urine. This is of great medical

Potassium (K⁺), Serum

significance when the patient is taking a potassium wasting diuretic without a potassium supplement or without potassium rich foods daily.

When acid-base balance is altered, the serum potassium also changes. As the pH of the blood increases (becomes more alkalotic) the potassium shifts from the serum to the cells. As the pH of the blood decreases (becomes more acidic) the intracellular potassium shifts to the serum. Clinical signs of hypokalemia include muscle weakness, cramps, hyporeflexia, paresthesias, decreased bowel motility, hypotension, cardiac arrhythmia, drowsiness, lethargy and coma. Serum potassium below 3.5 mEq/L is often seen with a serum pH above 7.45, decreased serum bicarbonate level and possibly elevated blood glucose.

Clinical signs of hyperkalemia include confusion, irritability, nausea, vomiting, intestinal colic, paresthesia abdominal cramps and muscle paralysis. Both hypokalemia and hyperkalemia can be life-threatening conditions requiring medical intervention.

Related Tests: sodium, serum, potassium, urine

Increased with:
- Renal failure
- Excessive intake or IV
- Cell damage:
  - burns
  - surgery
  - crushing injuries
  - chemotherapy

Decreased with:
- Malnutrition
- Malabsorption
- Diarrhea
- Severe vomiting
- Renal tubular acidosis
- Diuretic therapy
- Draining wounds

POTASSIUM (K+), SERUM

Increased with:
- Metabolic acidosis
- Addison's disease
- Internal hemorrhage
- Uncontrolled diabetes

- Sickle cell disease
- Hypoaldosteronism
- Hemolysis
- Dehydration
- Aldosterone inhibiting diuretics
- Infection
- Kidney transplant rejection
- Lupus erythematosus
- Interstitial nephritis

Decreased with:
- Chronic stress
- Chronic laxative abuse
- Cushing's syndrome
- IV fluids without adequate K+
- Alcoholism
- Deficient diet or IV intake
- Surgery
- Licorice ingestion
- Liver disease with ascites
- Hyperaldosteronism
- Renal artery stenosis
- Cystic fibrosis
- Trauma
- Chronic alcohol abuse
- Osmotic hyperglycemia
- Excessive sweating
- Bartter's syndrome
- Respiratory alkalosis
- Severe burns
- Barium chloride poisoning
- Vitamin B12 supplementation
- Folic acid supplementation

Medications that may increase levels:

ACE inhibitors	Aldesleukin	Amiloride
Aminocaproic acid	Aminoglutethimide	Ammonium chloride
Amphotericin B	Aripiprazole	Atenolol
Azathioprine	Azithromycin	Basiliximab
Benazepril	Betaxolol	Bisoprolol
Candesartan	Cannabis	Captopril
Cefdinir	Cefotaxime	Cisplatin
Clofibrate	Cyclosporine	Danazol
Dexamethasone	Digoxin	Doxorubicin
Enalapril	Eplerenone	Epoetin alfa
Erythropoietin	Etretinate	Felodipine
Fosphenytoin	Heparin	Indomethacin

POTASSIUM (K⁺), SERUM

Medications that may increase levels:

Isoniazid	Ketoconazole	Ketorolac
Labetalol	Lisinopril	Lithium
LMW heparin	Lovastatin	Mannitol
Methicillin	Methimazole	Methyltestosterone
Metoprolol	Micardis	Moexipril
Mycophenolate	Naproxen	Netilmicin
Nifedipine	Norfloxacin	NSIAD
Ofloxacin	Palonosetron	Paroxetine
Penicillamine	Penicillin	Pentamidine
Perindopril	Pindolol	Piroxicam
Potassium chloride	Procainamide	Propranolol
Quinapril	Quinupristin	Quinupristin/dalfopristin
Ramipril	Risedronate	Sirolimus
Somatropin	Spironolactone	Succinylcholine
Sulfamethoxazole	Sulindac	Tacrolimus
Timolol	Trandolapril	Triamterene
Trimethoprim	Tromethamine	Valsartan
Venlafaxine	Zalcitabine	

Medications that may decrease levels:

Acetazolamide	Albuterol	Aldesleukin
Aminosalicylic acid	Amlodipine	Ammonium chloride
Amphotericin	Arsenic trioxide	Aspirin
Azathioprine	Azithromycin	Basiliximab
Benzthiazide	Betamethasone	Betaxolol
Bevacizumab	Bisacodyl	Bortezomib
Bumetanide	Candesartan	Capreomycin
Captopril	Carbamazepine	Carbenicillin
Carvedilol	Cascara	Cathartics
Cephalexin	Chloroquine	Chlorothiazide
Chlorthalidone	Cidofovir	Cisplatin
Corticosteroids	Corticotropin	Cortisone
Dexamethasone	Digoxin	Diuretics
Dobutamine	Donepezil	Doxazosin
Doxorubicin	Enalapril	Epoprostenol
Ethacrynic acid	Etretinate	Felbamate
Fluconazole	Flucytosine	Fludrocortisone
Fluvoxamine	Formoterol	Foscarnet
Fosinopril	Fosphenytoin	Furosemide
Ganciclovir	Gentamicin	Glimepiride

POTASSIUM (K⁺), SERUM

Medications that may decrease levels:

Glucose	Hydrochlorothiazide	Imatinib
Indapamide	Insulin	Itraconazole
Ketoprofen	Laxatives	Levalbuterol
Levodopa	Lithium	Lomefloxacin
Methazolamide	Methyclothiazide	Methylprednisolone
Metoclopramide	Metolazone	Milrinone
Moricizine	Moxalactam	Mycophenolate
Nabumetone	Naproxen	Neomycin
Nifedipine	Nilutamide	Nisoldipine
Ondansetron	Pamidronate	Paroxetine
Penicillin	Pergolide	Piperacillin
Plicamycin	Polystyrene sulfonate	Polythiazide
Prednisolone	Prednisone	Quinethazone
Riluzole	Risperidone	Ritodrine
Sodium bicarbonate	Spironolactone	Streptozocin
Tacrolimus	Terbutaline	Tetracycline
Theophylline	Thiazides	Ticarcillin
Tobramycin	Triamterene	Trichlormethiazide
Trimethoprim	Venlafaxine	Vidarabine
Zalcitabine		

Potassium (K⁺), Urine

Normal Values 24 hr Urine
Child: 10-60 meq/L; 10-60 mmol/L (SI)
Adults: 25-125 meq/L; 25-125 mmol/L (SI)

Nutritional Significance

Potassium is an essential electrolyte that acts as part of the body's buffer system. Potassium balance is regulated in part by the kidneys. When serum potassium levels fall, the kidneys excrete less. It takes 1 to 3 weeks for the kidneys to conserve potassium effectively.

The urine potassium test requires a 24 hour urine collection to measure the total amount excreted. The data is useful in evaluating for renal, adrenal disorders and water and acid base imbalances. Urine potassium levels less than 20 mEq/L; 20 mmol/L are associated with nonrenal conditions. Values greater than 20 mEq/L; 20 mmol/L are associated with renal causes.

Urine potassium values are dependent upon diet. The transtubular potassium gradient (TTKG) is an index that reflects potassium conservation by the kidneys

TTKG= urine K/plasma K ÷ urine osm/plasma osm

Normal TTKG range with unrestricted diet = 8-9. TTKG levels greater than 10 are associated with high potassium diets and increased potassium excretion. TTKG levels less than 3 are associated with low potassium diets and less potassium excretion. TTKG levels less than 7 with hyperkalemia may indicate mineralocorticoid deficiency.

Related Tests: potassium, serum

POTASSIUM (K$^+$), URINE

Increased with:
- Renal failure
- Starvation (onset)
- Cushing's syndrome
- Diabetic acidosis
- Renal tubular acidosis
- Metabolic alkalosis
- Fanconi's syndrome
- Bartter's syndrome
- Aldosteronism

Decreased with:
- Addison's disease
- Pyelonephritis
- Glomerulonephritis

Medications that may increase levels:

Acetazolamide	Ammonia chloride	Antibiotics
Aspirin	Betamethasone	Bumetanide
Calcitonin	Carbenicillin	Cathartics
Chlorthalidone	Corticotropin	Cortisone
Corticosteroids	Dexamethasone	Diuretics
EDTA anticoagulant	Ethacrynic acid	Fenoldopam
Fludrocortisone	Gentamicin	Hydrochlorothiazide
Hydrocortisone	Indomethacin	Isosorbide
Levodopa	Licorice	Lithium
Mafenide	Methyclothiazide	Metolazone
Niacinamide	Oral contraceptives	Parathyroid extract
Penicillin	Prednisolone	Quinethazone
Streptozocin	Sulfates	Thiazides
Torsemide	Triamcinolone	Viomycin

Medications that may decrease levels:

Amiloride	Anesthetic agents	Carbamazepine
Cyclosporin A	Diazoxide	Felodipine
Ketoconazole	Levarterenol	Niacin
Ramipril	Sulfamethoxazole	Trimethoprim

Protein, Blood (Retinol Binding Protein, Prealbumin, Serum Albumin, Serum Globulin & Total Protein)

Retinol Binding Protein (RBP)
Normal Values
Adults: 2.6 – 7.6 mg/dL; 1.43-2.86 µmol/L(SI)

Nutritional Significance

RBP is a low molecular weight, single-chain polypeptide glycoprotein. It belongs to the α-globulin family of human plasma proteins and is the primary plasma transport protein for retinol. Once in circulation, the RBP-retinol complex binds to one molecule of transthyretin (prealbumin), a plasma thyroxine-binding protein. This complex then delivers retinol to specific receptors of the retina, skin, gonads, lungs, salivary glands and other tissues. RBP protects bound retinol from oxidation. It also regulates retinol release from the liver and mediates the specificity of its uptake by target cells.

RBP is a negative acute phase protein, meaning that levels plummet in the presence of acute or chronic inflammatory stress. An elevation in C-reactive protein (CRP) indicates acute inflammatory response. As the inflammatory process wanes, levels may rise, but it remains unclear if the changes reflect overall nutritional status. Research findings provide inconclusive data on whether RBP responds to protein and calorie restrictions or refeeding. RBP appears to be less affected by the acute inflammatory response than prealbumin or albumin possibly due to its short half-life. As long as CRP is elevated, RBP, prealbumin and albumin are significantly depressed. More studies are needed

Protein, Blood (Retinol Binding Protein, Prealbumin, Serum Albumin, Serum Globulin & Total Protein)

to determine the clinical significance of changes in RBP as inflammatory response wanes and as energy and protein intake increases.

RBP is not a reliable indicator of nutritional status in advanced chronic renal disease. All blood proteins increase in concentration in advanced kidney disease. These levels do not reflect the patient's protein status. RBP is not a reliable indicator of nutritional status in advanced liver disorders. The liver stores RBP and will release the stores as the liver disease progresses.

Immunoassays for serum levels of RBP are useful in the detection of liver disease and vitamin A deficiencies because vitamin A is important in the maintenance of differentiation and rate of proliferation of epithelial tissue. The determination of RBP serum levels have been shown to be important in the mediation of antitumor effects.

Related Tests: CRP, ESR, albumin, prealbumin

RBP Increased with:
- Advanced kidney disease
- Advanced liver disease

RBP Decreased with:
- Hyperthyroidism
- Chronic liver disorders
- Cystic fibrosis
- Zinc deficiency
- Sepsis
- Vitamin A deficiency
- Malnutrition
- Inflammatory disorders

Protein, Blood (Retinol Binding Protein, Prealbumin, Serum Albumin, Serum Globulin & Total Protein)

Prealbumin (PAB)
Normal Values

Newborn:	6-21 mg/dL; 60-210 mg/L (SI)
Child 1-5 yr:	14-30 mg/dL; 140-300 mg/L (SI)
Child 6-9 yr:	15-33 mg/dL; 150-330 mg/L (SI)
Child 10-13 yr:	22-36 mg/dL; 220-360 mg/L (SI)
Child 14-19 yr:	22-45 mg/dL; 220-450 mg/L (SI)
Adults:	15-36 mg/dL; 150-360 mg/L (SI)

Nutritional Significance

PAB is in a class of proteins having rapid turnover with short half-lives (2-3 days). PAB is also called transthyretin and thyroxine-binding prealbumin. It is secondary to thyroxine-binding globulin in the transportation of triiodothyronine (T3) and thyroxine (T4). PAB is a transport protein synthesized by the liver. It is transported in the serum as a complex of retinol-binding protein and vitamin A.

PAB is a negative acute phase protein, meaning that levels plummet in the presence of acute or chronic inflammatory stress. An elevation in C-reactive protein (CRP) indicates acute inflammatory response. As the inflammatory process wanes, levels may rise, but it remains unclear if the changes reflect overall nutritional status. Research findings provide inconclusive data on whether PAB responds to protein and calorie restrictions or refeeding. More studies are needed to determine the clinical significance of changes in PAB as inflammatory response wanes and as energy and protein intake increases.

Protein, Blood (Retinol Binding Protein, Prealbumin, Serum Albumin, Serum Globulin & Total Protein)

Related Tests: CRP, ESR, albumin, RBP, protein electrophoresis, immunoglobulin electrophoresis

PAB Increased with:
- Dehydration
- Nephrotic syndrome
- Hodgkin's disease
- Chronic kidney disease
- Pregnancy

PAB Decreased with:
- Overhydration
- Acute catabolic stress
- Malnutrition
- Liver damage
- Stress
- Salicylate poisoning
- Inflammation
- Infection
- Post-surgery
- AIDS
- Burns

Medications that may increase PAB levels:
Anabolic steroids   Androgens   Corticosteroids
Prednisolone

Medications that may decrease PAB levels:
Amiodarone   Estrogens   Oral contraceptives

PROTEIN, BLOOD (RETINOL BINDING PROTEIN, PREALBUMIN, SERUM ALBUMIN, SERUM GLOBULIN & TOTAL PROTEIN)

SERUM ALBUMIN
NORMAL VALUES

Premature infant:	3.0–4.2 g/dL; 30-42 g/L (SI)
Newborn:	3.5–5.4 g/dL; 35-54 g/L (SI)
Infant:	4.4–5.4 g/dL; 44-54 g/L (SI)
Child:	4.0–5.9 g/dL; 40-59 g/L (SI)
Adults:	3.5-5.0 g/dL; 35-50 g/L (SI)

NUTRITIONAL SIGNIFICANCE

Albumin, globulin and prealbumin constitute most of the protein within the body and are measured as total protein. Albumin is synthesized in the liver at a rate of 8 - 14 grams/day. It makes up approximately 60 percent of the total protein. Serum levels of albumin reflect hepatic cell function. When disease affects the liver cells, it loses its ability to synthesize albumin, prealbumin and globulin causing levels to diminish. Because of the long half-life (12-21 days) of albumin, severe impairments of the liver are not recognized quickly.

The major purpose of albumin is to maintain colloidal osmotic pressure. It also transports major blood constitutes, hormones, enzymes and medications. Albumin provides about 80 percent of colloidal osmotic pressure of the plasma. When serum albumin levels decrease, the water in plasma moves to the interstitial compartment. The end result is hypovolemia, which triggers renal retention of water and sodium. Albumin also serves as a carrier of metals, ions, fatty acids, amino acids,

PROTEIN, BLOOD (RETINOL BINDING PROTEIN, PREALBUMIN, SERUM ALBUMIN, SERUM GLOBULIN & TOTAL PROTEIN)

metabolites, bilirubin, enzymes, hormones and drugs.

Albumin is a negative acute phase protein, meaning that levels plummet in the presence of acute or chronic inflammatory stress. The albumin does not evaporate or disintegrate. It simply shifts from the extravascular space to the plasma. An elevation in C-reactive protein (CRP) indicates acute inflammatory response. As the inflammatory process wanes, levels may rise, but it remains unclear if the changes reflect overall nutritional status.

Levels of albumin may remain normal or near normal during uncomplicated starvation as redistribution from the interstitium to plasma occurs. For these reasons, a well-nourished patient may have low levels of the hepatic transport proteins, while a patient who has had significant weight loss and undernutrition may have normal or close to normal levels.

Another factor complicating the use of albumin for monitoring changes in nutrition status is related to the large extravascular albumin pool. Extravascular albumin concentration is 1.5 to 2 times higher than albumin in the blood. Some of the albumin pool returns to the circulation when blood concentrations decrease in non-stressed individuals, which tends to blunt changes in plasma albumin concentration. When the synthesis of albumin decreases, large amounts of albumin can return to the circulation. When synthesis of albumin increases, albumin leaves to replenish the extravascular pool.

PROTEIN, BLOOD (Retinol Binding Protein, Prealbumin, Serum Albumin, Serum Globulin and Total Protein)

Research findings provide inconclusive data on whether albumin responds to protein and calorie restrictions or refeeding. More studies are needed to determine the clinical significance of changes in albumin as inflammatory response wanes and as energy and protein intake increases.

When albumin levels are low the serum calcium level is also low. When the serum albumin is elevated the serum calcium is elevated. The reason for the interrelationship between albumin and calcium is that serum calcium levels represent both free calcium and calcium bound to albumin. When serum albumin levels are low, the ionized form of calcium is measured. This test is not affected by changes in serum albumin.

RELATED TESTS: CRP, ESR, PAB, RBP, protein electrophoresis, immunoglobulin electrophoresis

Albumin Increased with:
- Dehydration

Albumin Decreased with:
- Overhydration
- Inadequate oral intake
- Decreased absorption:
  - pancreatic insufficiency
  - malabsorption
- Impaired synthesis:
  - congestive heart failure
  - liver disease
  - acute stress

PROTEIN, BLOOD (RETINOL BINDING PROTEIN, PREALBUMIN, SERUM ALBUMIN, SERUM GLOBULIN & TOTAL PROTEIN)

Albumin Increased with:
Increased with:

Albumin Decreased with:
Decreased with:
- Increased need:
  - hyperthyroidism
  - pregnancy
- Increased loss:
  - edema
  - pressure ulcers
  - hemorrhage
  - nephrotic syndrome
  - Crohn's disease
  - sprue
  - Whipple's disease
  - AIDS
  - third-space losses:
  - burns
  - ascites
- Protein dilution secondary to excessive IV fluids
- Cushing's disease
- Thyrotoxicosis
- Increased capillary permeability
- Increased breakdown:
  - cancer
  - trauma
- Infection
- Inflammatory disease
- Familial idiopathic dysproteinemia

PROTEIN, BLOOD (RETINOL BINDING PROTEIN, PREALBUMIN, SERUM ALBUMIN, SERUM GLOBULIN & TOTAL PROTEIN)

Medications that may increase Albumin levels:

Anabolic steroids	Androgens	Corticosteroids
Dextran	Growth hormone	Insulin
Phenazopyridine	Prednisolone	Progesterone

Medications that may decrease Albumin levels:

Amiodarone	Ammonium ions	Estrogens
Hepatotoxic drugs	Oral contraceptives	

GLOBULIN
NORMAL VALUES
Adults: 2.3 - 3.4 g/dL; 23 - 34 g/L (SI)
Alpha1 globulin: 0.1-0.3 g/dL; 1-3 g/L(SI)
Alpha2 globulin: 0.6-1 g/dL; 6-10 g/L(SI)
Beta globulin: 0.7-1.1 g/dL; 7-11 g/L(SI)

NUTRITIONAL SIGNIFICANCE

Globulin makes up about 40 percent of the total protein. Globulin is synthesized in the reticuloendothelial system. It is the key building block of antibodies. While globulin can act as a transport vehicle, it does so to a lesser degree than albumin. It plays a lesser role than albumin in maintaining osmotic pressure.

Globulins are classified as alpha$_1$ globulin, alpha2 globulin and beta globulin. Alpha1 globulins transport proteins like thyroid and cortisol-binding globulin. The alpha2 globulins include serum haptoglobins, ceruloplasmin, prothrombin and cholinesterase. Beta globulins include lipoproteins, transferrin and plasminogen. Transferrin is increased in iron deficiency anemia and decreased

Protein, Blood (Retinol Binding Protein, Prealbumin, Serum Albumin, Serum Globulin & Total Protein)

in malnutrition. When both conditions are present, the levels may be within normal ranges.

Globulins are often normal or increased in diseases where albumin is depressed. For example, in lupus erythematosus the capillary permeability is increased. Since albumin is a smaller molecule than globulin, albumin is selectively lost into the extravascular space. In cases of liver disease, the liver may be unable to synthesize adequate levels of albumin, but the reticuloendothelial system can adequately produce globulin. This is seen in elderly individuals with compromised liver function.

Protein electrophoresis can separate various components of blood protein into bands or zones based on electrical charge. Several electrophoretic patterns have been identified and can be associated with specific diseases. See Table 23.

Related Tests: immunofixation electrophoresis, immunoglobulin electrophoresis, PAB

Globulin Increased with:
Alpha1
- Inflammatory disease

Alpha2
- Nephrotic syndrome
- Inflammatory disorders

Globulin Decreased with:
Alpha1
- Juvenile pulmonary emphysema

Alpha2
- Hemolysis
- Wilson's disease
- Hyperthyroidism
- Severe liver dysfunction

Protein, Blood (Retinol Binding Protein, Prealbumin, Serum Albumin, Serum Globulin & Total Protein)

Globulin Increased with:
Beta
- Hypercholesterolemia
- Iron deficiency anemia

Gamma globulin
- Multiple myeloma
- Waldenström's macroglobulinemia
- Chronic inflammatory disease
- Malignancy
- Acute and chronic infections

Globulin Decreased with:
Beta
- Malnutrition

Gamma globulin
- Genetic immune disorders
- Secondary immune deficiency

Total Protein
Normal Values

Premature infant:	4.2-7.6 g/dL; 42-76 g/L (SI)
Newborn:	4.6–7.4 g/dL; 46-74 g/L (SI)
Infant:	6.0-6.7 g/dL; 60-67 g/L (SI)
Child:	6.2-8.0 g/dL; 62-80 g/L (SI)
Adults:	6.4 - 8.3 g/dL; 64-83 g/L (SI)

Nutritional Significance

Total protein is a measure of the albumin, prealbumin and globulin in the blood. It is of little value as a sensitive index of protein intake and protein status.

Related Tests: PAB, RBP, albumin, globulin, protein electrophoresis, immunoglobulin electrophoresis

PROTEIN, BLOOD (RETINOL BINDING PROTEIN, PREALBUMIN, SERUM ALBUMIN, SERUM GLOBULIN & TOTAL PROTEIN)

TABLE 23. Protein Electrophoresis Patterns in Specific Diseases

Pattern	Electrophoresis	Diseases
Acute reaction	↓ albumin ↓ alpha2 globulin	acute infections, tissue necrosis, burns, surgery, stress, myocardial infarction
Chronic inflammation	slightly ↓ albumin ↓ gamma globulin ⇔ alpha2 globulin	chronic infections, granulomatous diseases, cirrhosis rheumatoid-collagen diseases
Nephrotic syndrome	↓↓ albumin ↑↑ alpha2 globulin ↑ ⇔ beta globulin	nephrotic syndrome
Advanced cirrhosis	↓ albumin ↑ gamma globulin Peaks of beta and gamma globulin	advanced cirrhosis
Polyclonal gamma globulin elevation	↑↑ gamma globulin with broad peak	cirrhosis, chronic infection, sarcoidosis, tuberculosis, endocarditis, rheumatoid-collagen diseases
Hypogammaglobulin-emia	↓ gamma globulin with other normal globulin levels	light-chain multiple myeloma
Monoclonal gammopathy	thin spikes in gamma globulin	myeloma, macroglobulinemia, gammopathies

Key: ↑ elevated, ↑↑ greatly elevated, ↓ decreased, ↓↓ greatly decreased, ⇔ Normal

Protein, Blood (Retinol Binding Protein, Prealbumin, Serum Albumin, Serum Globulin & Total Protein)

Total Protein
Increased with:
- Dehydration

Decreased with:
- Severe malnutrition
- Fluid overload
- Hepatic diseases
- AIDS
- Severe infection
- Protein-losing nephropathies
- Third-space losses
  - ascites
  - burns
- Lupus

PROTEIN, URINE (TOTAL PROTEIN, ALBUMIN, MICROALBUMIN)

NORMAL VALUES
TOTAL PROTEIN
Adults: None or up to 8 mg/dL
Adults: 50 - 80 mg/24 hr at rest
Adults: <250 mg/24 hr after strenuous exercise

ALBUMIN
Adults: <30 mg/24 hours

MICROALBUMIN
Adults: 0.2-1.9 mg/dL

MICROALBUMIN/CREATININE RATIO
Adults: 0-30 mg/g

NUTRITIONAL SIGNIFICANCE

A routine urinalysis includes evaluation for protein. Protein spilled into the urine is a sensitive indicator of kidney dysfunction. With normal kidney function little to no protein is found in the urine because the normal glomerular filtrate membranes are too small to allow protein through. However, in glomerulonephritis the spaces become larger and the protein can seep into the filtrate and into the urine. Loss of protein via the urine results in hypoproteinemia. This results in a decrease in normal capillary oncotic pressure that holds fluid within the vasculature. The combination of proteinuria and edema is called nephrotic syndrome.

Individuals with diabetes mellitus often develop renal complications. One early sign of this is microalbuminuria. This is

Protein, Urine (Total Protein, Albumin, Microalbumin)

a loss of greater than normal levels of albumin in the urine which is not detected in a routine urine testing. Excretion of 30 - 300 mg/ 24 hr of albumin is usually seen without a change in the glomerular filtration rate. The amount of albumin in the urine is a reflection of the duration of the diabetes and the glycemic control. Very high levels indicate the presence of diabetic nephropathy. Microalbuminuria can identify diabetic neuropathy about 5 years before routine protein tests. Diabetics with elevated microalbuminuria have a 5 to 10 fold increase in the occurrence of cardiovascular mortality, retinopathy and end stage kidney disease. A high percentage of these individuals will develop macroalbuminuria and excrete >300 mg/24 hours. This value indicates overt nephropathy and the glomerular filtration rate has declined significantly.

The presence of microalbuminuria in non-diabetics is an early indicator of lower life expectancy due to cardiovascular disease and hypertension.

Total Protein in Urine Increased with:
- Nephrotic syndrome
- Diabetes mellitus
- Multiple myeloma
- Preeclampsia, Toxemia
- Glomerulonephritis
- Congestive heart disease
- Malignant hypertension
- Polycystic disease
- Diabetic glomerulosclerosis
- Amyloidosis

PROTEIN, URINE (TOTAL PROTEIN, ALBUMIN, MICROALBUMIN)

Total Protein in Urine Increased with:
- Lupus erythematosus
- Goodpasture's syndrome
- Renal vein thrombosis
- Heavy-metal poisoning
- Galactosemia
- Bacterial pyelonephritis
- Nephrotoxic drug therapy
- Bladder tumors
- Acute infection
- Trauma, stress
- Leukemia
- Hyperthyroidism
- Renal transplant rejection
- Sickle cell
- Oxalosis

Albumin and Microalbumin in Urine Increased with:
- Glomerular damage
    - glomerulonephritis
    - lupus erythematosus
    - malignant hypertension
    - amyloidosis
    - nephrotic syndrome
    - polycystic kidney disease
- Diminished tubular resorption
    - renal tubular disease
    - cystinosis
    - Wilson's disease
    - Fanconi's syndrome
    - interstitial nephritis
- Diabetes mellitus
- Hypertension
- Cardiovascular disease
- Urinary bleeding
- Hemoglobinuria

Protein, Urine (Total Protein, Albumin, Microalbumin)

Albumin and Microalbumin in Urine Increased with:
- Myoglobinuria
- Pre-eclampsia

Medications that may increase levels:

Acetaminophen
Amikacin
Aminosalicylic acid
Arsenicals
Aspirin
Bacitracin
Betaxolol
Calcitriol
Carvedilol
Cefamandole
Cephalothin
Chloroform
Chlorpropamide
Cisplatin
Codeine
Corticotropin
Desipramine
Doxapram
Enalapril
Ergot preparations
Etretinate
Furosemide
Gentamicin
Griseofulvin
Ibuprofen
Interferon alfa-2a

Isoniazid
Ketorolac
Lithium
Mesalamine
Methicillin
Moxalactam
Nafcillin
Neomycin

Acetazolamide
Aminoglycosides
Amphotericin B
Ascorbic acid
Auranofin
Basiliximab
Bicarbonate
Capreomycin
Castor oil
Cefdinir
Chloral hydrate
Chlorpheniramine
Chlorthalidone
Clindamycin
Colistin
Cyclosporine
Diazoxide
Doxorubicin
Epirubicin
Ether
Fenoprofen
Gabapentin
Glyburide
Hepatitis A vaccine
Ifosfamide
Iodine-containing drugs
Isotretinoin
Lansoprazole
Mefenamic acid
Metaxalone
Mitomycin
Mycophenolate
Naphthalene
Nephrotoxic drugs

Aldesleukin
Aminophylline
Ampicillin
Asparaginase
Aurothioglucose
Benazepril
Bismuth subsalicylate
Carbamazepine
Cefaclor
Cephaloridine
Chlorhexidine
Chlorpromazine
Cidofovir
Clofibrate
Corticosteroids
Dantrolene
Dihydrotachysterol
Doxycycline
Eplerenone
Ethosuximide
Foscarnet
Gemcitabine
Glycerin
Hydralazine
Indomethacin
Iron

Kanamycin
Lipomul
Mercury compounds
Methenamine
Mitotane
Nabumetone
Naproxen
Netilmicin

PROTEIN, URINE (TOTAL PROTEIN, ALBUMIN, MICROALBUMIN)

Medications that may increase levels:

Nifedipine	Norfloxacin	NSAID
Ofloxacin	Olsalazine	Oxacillin
Oxaprozin	Paraldehyde	Paramethadione
Paromomycin	Penicillamine	Penicillin
Phenazopyridine	Phenolphthalein	Phosphorus
Piperacillin	Piroxicam	Plicamycin
Polymyxin B	Pregabalin	Probenecid
Promazine	Quinine	Radiographic agents
Ramipril	Ranitidine	Rifampin
Salicylates	Salsalate	Sevoflurane
Silver	Sodium bicarbonate	Sodium oxybate
Streptokinase	Sulfadiazine	Sulfamethoxazole
Sulfasalazine	Sulfisoxazole	Sulindac
Suprofen	Tacrolimus	Tegaserod
Tetracycline	Thallium	Theophylline
Thiabendazole	Ticarcillin	Ticlopidine
Tobramycin	Tolbutamide	Tolmetin
Tramadol	Triazolam	Trifluoperazine
Vancomycin	Venlafaxine	Verapamil
Zalcitabine		

Medications that may decrease levels:

Atenolol	Captopril	Cilostazol
Dipyridamole	Enalapril	Fosinopril
Furosemide	Ibuprofen	Indapamide
Perindopril	Quinapril	Ramipril

Prothrombin Time (PT) & International Normalized Ratio (INR)

Normal Values
Prothrombin Time 11-12.5 seconds
International Normalized Ratio 0.8-1.1

Nutritional Significance

PT is used to evaluate the adequacy of the common pathway for blood clotting. It measures the clotting ability of fibrinogen (factor I), prothrombin (factor II), factors V, VII and X. When these factors exist in insufficient qualities, the PT is prolonged. Clotting factors I, II, V, VII, IX and X are produced in the liver. In cirrhosis, hepatitis, the synthesis of these factors will not occur and serum concentrations decline. The synthesis of factors II, VII, IX and X are also dependent on vitamin K. In obstructive biliary disease, the bile required for fat absorption fails to enter the gut and fat soluble vitamins are not absorbed. While vitamin K can be synthesized in the gut, the malabsorption of dietary sources can contribute to lower levels of these clotting factors.

Anticoagulation medications warfarin and dicumarol are used to prevent coagulation in individuals with thromboembolic diseases. These medications interfere with the production of vitamin K dependent clotting factors which result in a prolonger PT time. The adequacy of anticoagulation medications can be monitored by following monitoring the PT or INR. The INR is a compared rating of PT ratios. The desirable INR for individuals

PROTHROMBIN TIME (PT) & INTERNATIONAL NORMALIZED RATIO (INR)

on anticoagulation therapy usually ranges between 2.0-3.0 for patients with atrial fibrillation and between 3.0-4.0 for patients with mechanical heart values. The ideal INR must be customized for each patient.

PT Increased with:
- Cirrhosis
- Hepatitis
- Vitamin K deficiency
- Excess alcohol intake
- Bile duct obstruction
- DIC
- Blood transfusion
- Deficiency of factors I, II, V, VII or X
- Hemorrhagic disease of newborn
- Fat malabsorption disorders
- Zollinger-Ellison syndrome

PT Decreased with:
- High fat diet
- High vitamin K intake
- Dehydration

Medications that may increase PT:
Allopurinol	Aminosalicylic acids	Antibiotica
Barbiturates	Beta-lactam	Cephalothins
Chloral hydrate	Chloramphenicol	Chloroprmazine
Cholestyramine	Cimetidine	Clofibrate
Coelstiol	Ethyl aocohol	Glucogon
Heparin	Methyldopa	Neomycin
Oral anticoagulatns	Propylthiouracil	Quinidine
Quinine	Salicylates	Sulfonamides

Medications that may decrease PT:
Anabolic steroids	Barbiturates	Chloral hydrate
Digitalis	Diphenhydramine	Estrogens
Griseofulvin	Oral contraceptives	Vitamin K

Red Blood Cell Indices (Mean Corpuscular Volume, Mean Corpuscular Hemoglobin, Mean Corpuscular Hemoglobin Concentration, Red Cell Distribution Width)

Nutritional Significance

The red blood cell indices are used to provide information about the size using MCV and RDW, weight using MCH and hemoglobin concentration of RBC using MCHC. These tests are part of a CBC and used to categorize anemias.

Mean Corpuscular Volume (MCV)
Normal Values

Newborn	96-108 μm^3; 96-108 fL (SI)
Child	80 - 95 μm^3; 80 - 95 fL (SI)
Adults:	80 - 95 μm^3; 80 - 95 fL (SI)

MCV is a measure of the average size or volume of a single RBC and is determined by dividing the hematocrit by the total RBC count.

$$MCV = \frac{\text{hematocrit (\%)} \times 10}{\text{RBC (million/mm}^3\text{)}}$$

When the MCV is increased, it suggests the RBC are macrocytic. Megaloblastic anemia (B12 & folic acid deficiency) are associated with an elevated MCV. A low MCV suggests the RBC are microcytic. Iron deficiency anemia and thalassemia are associated with decreased MCV.

Related Tests: CBC, HGB, HCT, MCH, MCHC, RDW

MCV Increased with:	**MCV Decreased with:**
■ Liver disease	■ Advanced iron deficiency
■ Folate deficiency	■ Chronic blood loss
■ B12 deficiency	■ Iron malabsorption

Red Blood Cell Indices (Mean Corpuscular Volume, Mean Corpuscular Hemoglobin, Mean Corpuscular Hemoglobin Concentration, Red Cell Distribution Width)

MCV Increased with:
- Excess alcohol intake
- Sprue and Celiac disease
- Early pernicious anemia
- Antimetabolite therapy
- Impaired absorption IF
- Gastrectomy
- Ileal resection
- Competitive parasites
- Hyperthyroidism
- Chronic pancreatic disease

MCV Decreased with:
- Excessive Fe
- Thalassemia
- Lead poisoning
- X-chromosome linked autosomal anemias

Mean Corpuscular Hemoglobin (MCH)
NORMAL VALUES

Newborn:	32-34 pg/cell
Child:	27 - 31 pg/cell
Adults:	27 - 31 pg/cell

MCH is a measure of the average weight of hemoglobin within a RBC. This value is determined by dividing the total hemoglobin concentration by the total number of RBC.

$$MCH = \frac{hemoglobin\ (g/dL) \times 10}{RBC\ (million/mm^3)}$$

Macrocytic cells tend to carry more hemoglobin than microcytic cells. The clinical implication is that MCH is generally elevated when there are macrocytic cells and depressed when there are microcytic cells.

RELATED TESTS: CBC, HGB, HCT, MCV, MCHC, RDW

Red Blood Cell Indices (Mean Corpuscular Volume, Mean Corpuscular Hemoglobin, Mean Corpuscular Hemoglobin Concentration, Red Cell Distribution Width)

MCH Increased with:
- Macrocytic anemia

MCH Decreased with:
- Microcytic anemia
- Fe anemia deficiency
- Hypochromic anemia
- Sickle cell anemia
- Hemolytic anemia
- Posthemorrhagic anemias

Mean Corpuscular Hemoglobin Concentration (MCHC)
Normal Values

Newborn	32-33 g/dL; 32%-33% (SI)
Child & Adults	32-36 g/dL; 32%-36% (SI)

MCHC is a measure of the average concentration of hemoglobin within a single RBC. It is derived by dividing the total hemoglobin concentration by the hematocrit.

$$MCHC = \frac{hemoglobin(g/dL) \times 100}{hematocrit(\%)}$$

Low levels of MCHC indicate that red blood cells have a deficiency of hemoglobin. These cells are described as hypochromic. When values are normal the cells are described as normocytic. MCHC is elevated in the presence of intravascular hemolysis because there is an increased concentration of hemoglobin in the blood. The automated counter records the free hemoglobin and incorporates it into the calculations. Cold agglutinins can cause a falsely high MCHC and MCV due to automated counter error.

Related Tests: CBC, HGB, HCT, MCH, MCV, RDW

Red Blood Cell Indices (Mean Corpuscular Volume, Mean Corpuscular Hemoglobin, Mean Corpuscular Hemoglobin Concentration, Red Cell Distribution Width)

MCHC Increased with:
- Spherocytosis
- Intravascular hemolysis
- Cold agglutinins

MCHC Decreased with:
- Iron deficiency
- Chronic blood loss
- Thalassemia

Red Cell Distribution Width (RDW)
NORMAL VALUES
Adults: 11-14.5%

RDW measures the variation of RBC size for classifying anemias. It is calculated by machine using MCV and RBC values. It is an indicator of the degree of anisocytosis, RBC of different and abnormal sizes. RDW is increased with macrocytic anemias because there is fragmentation of macrocytic cells. In sickle cell anemia, there is increased RDW variation due to the abnormal size of the cells and different amounts of hemoglobin. With post-hemorrhagic anemias, the RDW is elevated because the bone marrow's response to bleeding is to release premature RBCs into the blood stream which are. larger than mature RBCs and contribute to RDW variation.

RELATED TESTS: CBC, HGB, HCT, MCV, MCH, MCHC

RDW Increased with:
- Iron deficiency
- Macrocytic anemia
- Sickle cell disease
- Hemolytic anemias
- Posthemorrhagic anemias

RETICULOCYTE COUNT (RETIC COUNT), RETICULOCYTE INDEX

NORMAL VALUES
RETICULOCYTE COUNT
Newborn	2.5%-6.5% of total number RBCs
Infant	0.5%-3.1% of total number RBCs
Child	0.5% - 2% of total number RBCs
Adults:	0.5%-2% of total number RBCs

RETICULOCYTE INDEX
Adults   1.0

NUTRITIONAL SIGNIFICANCE

A reticulocyte is an immature red blood cell, typically comprising about 1 to 2 percent of the RBC in the human body. Reticulocytes develop and mature in the bone marrow. They are called reticulocytes because of a reticular (mesh-like) network of RNA that becomes visible under a microscope with certain stains. Reticulocytes are slightly larger than healthy mature RBC.

Reticulocytes circulate in the bloodstream for about 2 days before developing into mature RBC. The reticulocyte count increases during rapid blood loss or in the course of certain diseases in which RBC are destroyed prematurely. Also, patients living at high elevations may have increased reticulocyte counts as one way to compensate for the lower oxygen levels found at high altitudes.

The reticulocyte count is an indication of the ability of the bone marrow to responds to anemia and produce healthy RBC. It evaluates for both bone marrow function and erythropoietic activity. It is a percentage of the total number of RBCs and is used

RETICULOCYTE COUNT (RETIC COUNT), RETICULOCYTE INDEX

to classify anemias.

A normal or low reticulocyte count in a patient with anemia indicates that the bone marrow is unable to produce enough RBC. An elevated reticulocyte count in a patient with a normal hemoglobin indicates normal RBC production compensating for an ongoing loss of RBC. The patient with anemia is expected to have a low reticulocyte count. However, since the reticulocyte count is a percentage of total RBC, the level may appear elevated because the total number of mature RBC is low. One way to evaluate the reticulocyte count in a patient with anemia is to determine the reticulocyte index.

$$\text{Reticulocyte index} = \text{retic count (\%)} \times \frac{\text{Patient's hematocrit}}{\text{Normal hematocrit}}$$

The reticulocyte index in a patient with an adequate bone marrow response is expected to be 1.0. If the value is less than 1.0, this suggests the bone marrow response is inadequate even though the reticulocyte count is elevated. Reticulocyte index values less than 2 percent indicates hypoproliferative component of anemia. Values greater than 2-3 percent suggests increased RBC production.

RELATED TESTS: CBC, HGB, HCT, MCV

Increased with:
- Hemolytic anemia
- Hemorrhage
- Erythroblastosis fetalis

Decreased with:
- Iron deficiency
- Pernicious anemia
- Megaloblastic anemia

Reticulocyte Count (Retic Count), Reticulocyte Index

Increased with:
- Postsplenectomy
- Treatment for nutritional anemias
- Leukemias
- Sickle cell anemia
- RBC enzyme deficits
- Pregnancy
- Malaria

Decreased with:
- Aplastic anemia
- Anemia of chronic & inflammatory diseases
- Radiation therapy
- Malignancy
- Myelodysplastic syndromes
- Chronic infection
- Bone marrow failure
- Anterior pituitary hypofunction
- Adrenocortical insufficiency
- Cirrhosis
- Alcoholism

SCHILLING TEST; VITAMIN B12 ABSORPTION TEST

NORMAL VALUES
Adults: 8-40% of radioactive B12 excreted within 24 hrs

NUTRITIONAL SIGNIFICANCE

Use of the Schilling test for detection of pernicious anemia has been supplanted for the most part by serologic testing for parietal cell and intrinsic factor antibodies. Other effective biomarkers of a change in vitamin B12 intake include plasma and serum concentrations of total vitamin B12, methylmalonic acid, and total homocysteine. One promising test reported in the scientific literature is plasma holotranscobalamin.

The Schilling test maybe used when the folate levels are elevated suggesting a B12 deficiency or pernicious anemia or when clinical symptoms suggest a B12 deficiency. It evaluates the body's ability to absorb B_{12} given orally, but does not evaluate B12 stores.

A lack of dietary B12 or an under utilization of B12 usually causes pernicious anemia. The most common etiology of pernicious anemia is due to a gastric mucosa defect resulting in inadequate secretion of intrinsic factor. When B12 is ingested it combines with intrinsic factor (IF) and is absorbed in the distal part of the ileum. Without IF, B12 can not be absorbed, body stores are depleted and the body produces enlarged immature red blood cells.

The Schilling test evaluates the body's ability to absorb B12. With normal absorption, the ileum absorbs more vitamin B12

SCHILLING TEST; VITAMIN B_{12} ABSORPTION TEST

than needed. The excess is excreted in the urine. When absorption is impaired, there are minimal amounts of B12 excreted in the urine. The Schilling test includes two stages, stage one includes an oral radioactive dose of B12 alone. A 24-48 hour urine collection for B12 is obtained. If the excretion of radioactive B12 metabolites is less than 8 percent, it appears that IF is lacking or there is a malabsorption problem. Next, a stage two test is done. This time the patient is given an oral radioactive dose of B12 combined with human IF. If stage two results are normal this suggests IF is inadequate. However, if stage two results are abnormal this suggests a malabsorption problem.

      A combined one-stage - two-stage Schilling test is also used. The patient receives one dose of cobalt-57 labeled B12 plus IF and a dose of cobalt-58 labeled B12. Urine is collected for 24-48 hours. The percentages of cobalt-57 and cobalt-58 are determined. With pernicious anemia secondary to inadequate IF only the cobalt-57 labeled B12 will be excreted. However, if the pernicious anemia is caused by primary bowel malabsorption then no radioactive B12 metabolites will be present in the urine. Elderly patients, those with renal insufficiency, diabetes or hypothyroidism may have reduced excretion of vitamin B12. Patients are advised not to take laxatives during the test because they could decrease the rate of vitamin B12 absorption.

SCHILLING TEST; VITAMIN B_{12} ABSORPTION TEST

The Schilling test is also helpful in confirming a diagnosis of intestinal bacteria overgrowth in the small bowel. The results of the stage one and stage two Schilling tests are often abnormal. However, with antibiotic treatment the results of a repeated Schilling tests are normal.

RELATED TESTS: vitamin B12, IF antibodies

Decreased with:
- Pernicious anemia
- Intestinal malabsorption
- Hypothyroidism
- Liver disease
- Regional enteritis
- Lymphomas
- Blind loop syndrome
- Scleroderma
- Small bowel diverticula
- Crohn's disease

Medications that may increase levels:
Chloral hydrate   Omeprazole

Medications that may decrease levels:
Anticonvulsants	Ascorbic acid	Chlorpromazine
Cholestyramine	Colchicine	Laxatives
Metformin	Neomycin	Octreotide
Oral contraceptives	Ranitidine	Rifampin

SODIUM (Na⁺), SERUM

NORMAL VALUES
Newborn	134-144 mEq/L; 134-144 mmol/L (SI)
Infant	134-150 mEq/L; 134-150 mmol/L (SI)
Child	136-145 mEq/L; 136-145 mmol/L (SI)
Adults:	136-145 mEq/L; 136-145 mmol/L (SI)

NUTRITIONAL SIGNIFICANCE

Sodium is the major cation in extracellular space. The concentration of sodium between cells is approximately 140 mEq/L compared to 5 mEq/L within the cells. The serum sodium level reflects the relationship between total body sodium and extracellular fluid volume. The concentration of sodium serves as a major determinant of extracellular osmolality. The serum sodium level reflects the balance between dietary intake and renal excretory function. As free body water increases, the serum sodium level decreases. The kidneys respond by conserving sodium and excreting water. However, if the free body water decreases, the serum sodium increases, then the kidneys conserve water.

Approximately 90 to 250 mEq/day of sodium is required to maintain sodium balance in adults. The healthy kidney can excrete about 450-500 mEq of sodium per day. If an individual without normal diuresis or prior sodium deficit, consumes more than that amount, the serum levels will probably increase. Factors which regulate sodium balance include aldosterone, natriuretic

Sodium (Na⁺), Serum

hormone and ADH. When the sodium level in the extracellular fluid is decreased, the adrenal glands secrete aldosterone which stimulates reabsorption by the kidneys. A decreased serum sodium level also results in a decreased extracellular osmolality.

When the extracellular fluid sodium level is within normal range aldosterone secretion is decreased, which allows for sodium excretion. However, if the extracellular fluid level of sodium exceeds the normal limits there is an increased extracellular osmolality. The elevated osmolality stimulates secretion of the ADH, which in turn increases tubular reabsorption of water. Natriuretic hormone also promotes excretion of sodium. Diseases that increase aldosterone secretion such as Cushing's disease and hyperaldosteronism stimulate the kidney to reabsorb sodium at the renal tubule. Diseases associated with a deficiency of ADH such as diabetes insipidus, will have large fluid losses and sodium levels become concentrated. Clinical signs of hypernatremia include dehydration, thirst, agitation, restlessness, hyperreflexia, mania, tachycardia, dry mucous membranes, lethargy, hyperactive reflexes and seizures. Serum levels greater than 152 mEq/L; 152 mmol/L are associated with cardiovascular and renal symptoms. Levels greater than 160 mEq/L; 160 mmol/can cause heart failure. As the fluid shifts to compensate for excessive levels of sodium the serum becomes more dilute. Other laboratory values associated

Sodium (Na⁺), Serum

with hypernatremia include urine specific gravity greater than 1.015 and serum osmolality greater than 295 mOsm/kg H2O.

All laboratory values will appear less concentrated when hyponatremia is present. The body compensates for hyponatremia by increasing water loss. As water is lost, the serum sodium becomes more concentrated as well as other laboratory values. Serum levels less than 125 mEq/L; 125 mmol/L are associated with weakness and dehydration. Levels ranging from 90-105 mEq/L; 90-105 mmol/can result in severe neurologic symptoms and vascular problems. Other laboratory values associated with hyponatremia include urine specific gravity less than 1.010 and serum osmolality greater than 285 mOsm/kg H2O. Diseases associated with a deficiency of aldosterone, such as Addison's disease, will experience hyponatremia because sodium is not reabsorbed by the kidneys. Syndrome of inappropriate antidiuretic hormone (SIADH) secretion results in hyponatremia because the oversecretion of ADH stimulates the kidney to reabsorb free water and ultimately dilutes serum sodium levels. Other disorders associated with fluid retention and sodium dilution include ascites, peripheral edema, pleural effusion and congestive heart failure. Clinical signs of hyponatremia include muscle cramps and twitching, headache, dizziness, lethargy, confusion, convulsions, stupor and coma. The changes in the central nervous system are due to fluid shifts from the

Sodium (Na$^+$), Serum

extracellular spaces to the intracellular spaces and cause the cells to swell. Elevated blood glucose levels give falsely low serum sodium values. Reasons that serum sodium levels are low include:
- The osmotically active glucose draws water from cells into intravascular space creating a dilution effect.
- Dehydration stimulates increased water retention creating a dilution effect.
- Severe hypertriglyceridemia with metabolic decompensation may displace some of the aqueous component of the blood and sodium is only found in the aqueous component.

Related Tests: urine sodium, aldosterone, ADH

Increased with:
- Increased Na intake:
  - excessive Na in IV fluids
  - excessive Na intake
- Excessive free body loss:
  - dehydration
  - excessive sweating
- Excessive free body loss:
  - diabetes insipidus
  - osmotic diuresis
  - thermal burns
  - GI losses without rehydration
- Decreased Na losses:
  - Cushing's syndrome
- Hyperaldosteronism

Decreased with
- Decreased Na intake:
  - deficient diet
  - deficient Na in IV fluids
- Excessive free sodium loss:
  - Addison's disease
  - diarrhea or vomiting
- Excessive free sodium loss:
  - intraluminal bowel loss
  - diuretic therapy
  - chronic renal insufficiency
  - large volume aspiration of pleural or peritoneal fluid
- Third-space losses
  - ascites
  - pleural effusion
  - ileus or obstruction

SODIUM (Na⁺), SERUM

Decreased with
- Increased free body water
  - excessive oral water intake
  - hyperglycemia
  - SIADH
  - excessive IV fluid intake
  - congestive heart failure
  - peripheral edema
  - osmotic dilution
- Nephrotic syndrome
- Pyloric obstruction
- Malabsorption syndrome
- Diabetic acidosis
- Water intoxication
- Hypothyroidism

Medications that may increase levels:

Aldesleukin	Amiloride	Amino acids
Ampicillin	Anabolic steroids	Betamethasone
Cannabis	Carbamazepine	Carbenicillin
Cefotaxime	Chlorthalidone	Cholestyramine
Clonidine	Corticosteroids	Cortisone
Diazoxide	Doxorubicin	Estrogens
Etretinate	Fludrocortisone	Fosphenytoin
Growth Hormone	Guanethidine	Hydrocortisone
Isosorbide	Ketoprofen	Mannitol
Methyclothiazide	Methyldopa	Methyltestosterone
Nitrofurantoin	Oral contraceptives	Penicillin G
Phenelzine	Polystyrene sulfonate	Prednisolone
Prednisone	Progesterone	Ramipril
Sildenafil	Sodium bicarbonate	Sodium phenylbutyrate
Sodium sulfate	Tetracycline	Ticarcillin/clavulanate
Valproic acid	Vitamin E	Zalcitabine

Sodium (Na$^+$), Serum

Medications that may decrease levels:

Acetaminophen	Acetazolamide	Amiloride
Aminoglutethimide	Ammonium chloride	Amphotericin
Atovaquone	Benazepril	Captopril
Carbamazepine	Carvedilol	Cathartics
Chlorothiazide	Chlorpropamide	Chlorthalidone
Cisplatin	Clofibrate	Clonidine
Clozapine	Cyclophosphamide	Cytarabine
Dapsone	Desmopressin	Diclofenac
Diuretics	Doxepin	Doxorubicin
Doxycycline	Eplerenone	Esomeprazole
Ethacrynic acid	Etretinate	Fluoxetine
Fluvoxamine	Foscarnet	Furosemide
Gentamicin	Glimepiride	Glyburide
Glycerin	Haloperidol	Hydrochlorothiazide
Hydroflumethiazide	Indomethacin	Isosorbide dinitrate
Itraconazole	Ketoconazole	Ketoprofen
Ketorolac	Laxatives	Lisinopril
Lithium	Mannitol	Methyclothiazide
Methylprednisolone	Metolazone	Miconazole
Morphine	Nicardipine	Nifedipine
Nisoldipine	Nitrofurantoin	NSAID
Olanzapine	Omeprazole	Oxycodone
Oxytocin	Paroxetine	Pentostatin
Phenoxybenzamine	Pimozide	Polythiazide
Pralidoxime	Pravastatin	Propafenone
Quinethazone	Ramipril	Riluzole
Risperidone	Sertraline	Sirolimus
Sodium bicarbonate	Somatostatin	Spironolactone
Sulfonylureas	Tacrolimus	Theophylline
Thiazides	Ticlopidine	Tobramycin
Trastuzumab	Trimethoprim	Trimetrexate
Trimipramine	Trovafloxacin	Valproic acid
Vasopressin	Venlafaxine	Vidarabine
Vincristine	Zalcitabine	

Sodium (Na⁺), Urine

Normal Values
Adults: 40-220 mEq/day; 40-220 mmol/day (SI)

Nutritional Significance
The sodium content of the urine reflects the balance between dietary intake and the renal excretion of sodium. In a healthy individual, nonrenal sodium losses are minimal. Many factors affect the homeostatic sodium balance. Aldosterone secretion decreases urine sodium levels by stimulating conservation of sodium. ADH secretion increases resorption of water in the distal tubules of the kidney and increases urine sodium levels.

The urine sodium test evaluates the total sodium excreted in urine over 24 hours. Measuring the amount of sodium excreted is useful in evaluating patients with volume depletion, acute renal failure, adrenal disturbances and acid-base imbalances. The results of this test are helpful to assess the patient with a low serum sodium level.

Related Tests: serum sodium, aldosterone, ADH

Increased with:	**Decreased with:**
■ Dehydration	■ Congestive heart failure
■ Hypothyroidism	■ Malabsorption
■ Toxemia of pregnancy	■ Inadequate Na intakes
■ Diuretic therapy	■ Cushing's syndrome
■ Diabetic ketoacidosis	■ Aldosteronism
■ SIADH	■ Diaphoresis
■ Salt-losing nephritis	■ Pulmonary emphysema

SODIUM (Na+), URINE

Increased with:
- Adrenocortical insufficiency
- Addison's disease
- Tubulointerstitial disease
- Bartter's syndrome

Decreased with:
- Nephrotic syndromes with acute oliguria
- Prerenal azotemia

Medications that may increase levels:

ACE inhibitors	Acetazolamide	Amiloride
Ammonium chloride	Aspirin	Atenolol
Benzthiazide	Bumetanide	Calcitonin
Captopril	Carvedilol	Chlorothiazide
Chlorthalidone	Cisplatin	Clofibrate
Cyclothiazide	Dexamethasone	Digitalis
Doxepin	Enalapril	Ethacrynic acid
Felodipine	Fenoldopam	Furosemide
Hydrochlorothiazide	Hydrocortisone	Hydroflumethiazide
Ifosfamide	Indomethacin	Insulin
Isosorbide	Levodopa	Lithium
Losartan	Mannitol	Methyclothiazide
Metoprolol	Metolazone	Niacin
Niacinamide	Oral contraceptives	Paramethasone
Parathyroid extract	Polythiazide	Progesterone
Quinethazone	Secretin	Spironolactone
Tetracycline	Thiazides	Torsemide
Triamcinolone	Triamterene	Trichlormethiazide
Trimethoprim	Verapamil	Vincristine

Medications that may decrease levels:

Anesthetic agents	Carbamazepine	Corticosteroids
Cortisone	Cyclosporine	Diazoxide
Etodolac	Fluoxetine	Ibuprofen
Indomethacin	Insulin	Ketorolac
Levarterenol	Lithium	Methylprednisolone
Naproxen	Nifedipine	Octreotide
Omeprazole	Propranolol	Ramipril

SPECIFIC GRAVITY, URINE

NORMAL VALUES
Adults: 1.005-1.030
Elderly: values decrease with age

NUTRITIONAL SIGNIFICANCE

Specific gravity measures the concentration of particles, wastes and electrolytes, in urine. The measurement is the weight of the urine compared to distilled water (specific gravity = 1.000.) A high specific gravity indicates concentrated urine. A low specific gravity indicates dilute urine. It is used to evaluate the excretory and concentrating power of the kidneys. Renal disease and age tend to reduce the kidney's ability to concentrate urine resulting in a low specific gravity. Specific gravity must be interpreted in conjunction with other laboratory test results. The presence of glucose and protein in the urine will increase the specific gravity. It is a measurement of hydration status. The edematous patient will have a more dilute urine with a lower specific gravity. The dehydrated patient will have an abnormally high specific gravity. Specific gravity correlates roughly with osmolality. It is usually evaluated using a refractometer or dipstick.

RELATED TESTS: urine osmolality

Increased with:
- Dehydration
- Diabetes mellitus
- Fever
- Vomiting
- Congestive heart failure
- Toxemia of pregnancy
- Diarrhea

Decreased with:
- Early chronic renal disease
- Severe renal damage
- Diabetes insipidus
- Glomerulonephritis
- Edema
- Aging

Thiamin (B1)

Normal Values, Whole Blood
Adults: 80-150 nmol/L(SI)

Nutritional Significance

Thiamin is a water soluble vitamin absorbed in the proximal jejunum by active transport. Body tissues store about 30 mg but use about 1-2 mg daily. It has a half-life of 9-18 days. Thiamine pyrophosphate is essential for the proper transfer of the aldehyde groups, and it is an essential coenzyme for glycolytic and pentose pathways of glucose metabolism. Enzymes that require thiamine include pyruvate dehydrogenase, α-ketoglutarate dehydrogenase, transketolase, and branched-chain α-ketoacid dehydrogenase.

Persistent vomiting, a deficient diet or excessive utilization can deplete thiamin rapidly. Glucose infusions given to a patient with depleted thiamin status will worsen symptoms and may cause permanent cognitive and neuromuscular impairments.

Primary thiamin deficiency is caused by inadequate intake (e.g. diet of highly refined carbohydrates). Secondary thiamin deficiency is caused by increased demand, impaired absorption, or impaired metabolism. In alcoholics, thiamin deficiency may occur due to decreased intake, impaired absorption, increased demand, and possibly an apoenzyme defect.

Thiamin deficiency can cause wet beriberi or dry beriberi. Congestive heart failure is the primary symptom of wet beriberi.

THIAMIN (B1)

The first effects are vasodilation, tachycardia, a wide pulse pressure, sweating, warm skin and lactic acidosis. Later, heart failure develops, causing orthopnea and pulmonary and peripheral edema. Vasodilation can continue, sometimes resulting in shock.

Dry beriberi refers to peripheral neurologic deficits due to thiamin deficiency. These deficits affect predominantly the lower extremities, beginning with paresthesias in the toes, burning in the feet, heaviness in legs, muscle cramps and tenderness in the calves, difficulty rising from a squatting position, and decreased vibratory sensation in the toes, and plantar dysesthesias are early signs. As beriberi progresses hair loss, muscle wasting and severe burning in feet are seen.

Wernicke-Korsakoff syndrome occurs in some alcoholics who do not consume foods fortified with thiamin. Wernicke's encephalopathy consists of psychomotor slowing or apathy, nystagmus, ataxia, ophthalmoplegia, impaired consciousness, and, if untreated, coma and death. Korsakoff's psychosis consists of mental confusion, dysphonia, and confabulation with impaired memory of recent events.

Plasma and serum levels of thiamin reflect recent dietary changes and may be misleading. The most appropriate way to measure thiamin status is to measure thiamin diphosphate in whole blood. Also a pyruvate level of >1 mg/dL is a reliable indicator of deficiency and erythrocyte transketolase activity of <0.017 U/dL indicates deficiency.

THIAMIN (B1)

Increased with:
- Supplemental thiamin

Decreased with:
- Deficient diet
- Hyperthyroidism
- Prolonged vomiting
- Prolonged diarrhea
- Malabsorption syndromes
- Bariatric procedures
- Alcoholism
- Hepatic insufficiency

THYROID FUNCTION TESTS (THYROID-STIMULATING HORMONE (TSH), THYROTROPIN-RELEASING HORMONE (TRH), THYROXINE-BINDING GLOBULIN (TBG), THYROXINE (T4), FREE THYROXINE (T4), FREE THYROXINE INDEX (FTI), TRIIODOTHYRONINE (T3), FREE TRIIODOTHYRONINE (FREE T3)

NUTRITIONAL SIGNIFICANCE

The thyroid is a butterfly-shaped gland that lies in front the trachea, just below the larynx. It is unique among endocrine glands because it has a large store of hormone and a slow rate of turnonver. Thyroxine (T4) and triiodothyronine (T3) are produced by the thyroid gland when the anterior pituitary gland releases thyroid-stimulating hormone (TSH).

These hormones are produced when tyrosine combines with iodine to form monoiodotyrosine. The complex binds with an additional iodine to form diiodotyrosine. Two diiodotyrosine molecules combine to form tetraiodothyronine or T4. If a diiodotyrosine molecule combines with a monoiodotyrosine, triiodothyronine or T3 is formed. However, a significant proportion of T3 is formed in the liver by conversion of T4 to T3. T3 is less stable than T4 because it is less tightly bound to serum proteins.

Laboratory tests are ordered to distinguish between normal thyroid function or euthyroidism, increased thyroid function or hyperthyroidism and decreased function or hypothyroidism. It is estimated that approximately 5 percent of adult women and 3 percent of adult men have subclinical thyroid disease. The prevalence increases with age and is greater in

THYROID FUNCTION TESTS (THYROID-STIMULATING HORMONE (TSH), THYROTROPIN-RELEASING HORMONE (TRH), THYROXINE-BINDING GLOBULIN (TBG), THYROXINE (T_4), FREE THYROXINE (T_4), FREE THYROXINE INDEX (FTI), TRIIODOTHYRONINE (T_3), FREE TRIIODOTHYRONINE (FREE T_3)

Caucasians than in African-Americans. Untreated hypothyroidism can lead to fatigue, weight gain, mental slowing, heart failure and elevated lipid levels. Subclinical hyperthyroidism occurs in 1 percent of men over age 60 and 1.5 percent of women over age 60. Patients with hypothyroidism often develop dyspnea on exertion, fatigue, bradycardia and edema that may be the result of either pericardial effusion or congestive heart failure. Patients also have an increased incidence of hypercholesterolemia and hypertriglyceridemia. Patients have an increased LDL, VLDL, HDL, Apo B-71, and Lp[a]. Thyroid hormone replacement therapy typically improves their lipid profiles. Both symptomatic and subclinical hypothyroidism may be risk factors for premature CAD and hypertension.

Untreated hyperthyroidism can lead to atrial fibrillation, congestive heart failure, osteoporosis, arterial thromboembolism, hypertension and neuropsychiatric problems. Mitral valve prolapse syndromes are more common in women with Graves' disease. Also, hyperthyroid patients can present with angina symptoms in the absence of coronary artery disease. Symptoms may be improved with treatment for thyroid disease.

Total T4, total T3, Free Thyroxine Index (FTI) and TSH are the most useful test to confirm or exclude hyperthyroidism.

Thyroid Function Tests (Thyroid-Stimulating Hormone (TSH), Thyrotropin-Releasing Hormone (TRH), Thyroxine-Binding Globulin (TBG), Thyroxine (T4), Free Thyroxine (T4), Free Thyroxine Index (FTI), Triiodothyronine (T3), Free Triiodothyronine (Free T3)

The most useful tests to confirm or exclude hypothyroidism are total T4, FTI, and TSH. Typical pattern of results for thyroid dysfunction is noted on Table 24. Each test is discussed in detail in the next section.

Table 24. Pattern of Test Results for Thyroid Dysfunction

Lab test	Hyperthyroidism	Hypothyroidism
thyroxine (T4)	↑	↓
triiodothyronine (T3)	↑	↓
free T4 (f T4)	↑	↓
free T3 (f T3)	↑	↓
thyroid stimulating hormone (TSH)	↓	↑
thyroid releasing hormone (TRH)	↓	↑
free thyroxine index (FTI)	↑	↓

Thyroid Stimulating Hormone (TSH)
Normal Values
Newborn:	3-18 µU/mL; 3-18 mU/L (SI)
Cord:	2-10 µU/mL; 2-10 mU/L (SI)
Adults:	3-12 µU/mL; 3-12 mU/L (SI)

Values vary among laboratories.

Nutritional Significance

Low levels of T3 and T4 stimulate the hypothalamus to release thyroid-releasing hormone (TRH). TRH acts on the anterior pituitary gland to secrete TSH, also called thyrotropin.

Thyroid Function Tests (Thyroid-Stimulating Hormone (TSH), Thyrotropin-Releasing Hormone (TRH), Thyroxine-Binding Globulin (TBG), Thyroxine (T4), Free Thyroxine (T4), Free Thyroxine Index (FTI), Triiodothyronine (T3), Free Triiodothyronine (Free T3)

TRH is also called thyrotropin-releasing hormone. TSH level is elevated in hypothyroidism and reduced in hyperthyroidism because the high levels of thyroid hormones inhibits the release of TSH. It is the single most sensitive test for primary hypothyroidism. If there is evidence of hypothyroidism, but the TSH is not elevated, hypopituitarism may be present.

The concentration of TSH is useful in differentiating primary from secondary hypothyroidism. There is a compensatory increase of TRH and TSH in individuals with primary hypothyroidism. Examples of primary hypothyroidism include surgical or radioactive ablation, burned-out thyroiditis, thyroid agnesis, idiopathic hypothyroidism or congenital cretinism and in patients taking anti-thyroid medications. In secondary hypothyroidism, the function of the pituitary gland is faulty due to a tumor, trauma or infarction. Diseases of the anterior pituitary diminish the production of TSH. In tertiary hypothyroidism, the function of the hypothalamus is faulty due to tumor, trauma or infarction. Diseases of the hypothalamus diminish the capability of the hypothalamus to secrete TRH, which in turn reduces TSH production and secretion. In either secondary or tertiary hypothyroidism there are low levels of T3 and T4.

TSH test is used to monitor exogenous thyroid

Thyroid Function Tests (Thyroid-Stimulating Hormone (TSH), Thyrotropin-Releasing Hormone (TRH), Thyroxine-Binding Globulin (TBG), Thyroxine (T4), Free Thyroxine (T4), Free Thyroxine Index (FTI), Triiodothyronine (T3), Free Triiodothyronine (Free T3)

replacement or thyroid suppression. The goal of replacement therapy is to provide a euthyroid state and of suppression therapy is to completely suppress the thyroid gland and TSH secretion via excessive medication. Suppression therapy may be helpful to reduce the size of a thyroid goiter. Individuals with severe, chronic diseases may have increased levels of TSH, in which low levels of thyroid hormone act as a stimulant to release TSH from the anterior pituitary. In some cases, the TSH level may decline.

TSH measurements with sufficient sensitivity to distinguish between low levels and normal levels are the preferred test to diagnose hyperthyroidism. However, the high sensitivity TSH test is used to diagnose patients with sick euthyroid and to distinguish between mild hyperthyroidism and Graves' disease.

TSH Increased with:
- Primary hypothyroidism
- Hashimoto's thyroiditis
- Thyroid agenesis
- Thyrotropin-producing tumors
- Thyrotoxicosis due to pituitary tumor
- Hypothyroid patients receiving inadequate thyroid replacement hormone

TSH Decreased with:
- Primary hyperthyroidism
- Factitious hyperthyroidism
- Euthyroidism sick disease
- Secondary hypothyroidism
- Suppressive doses of thyroid medication

Medications that may increase TSH levels:

Amiodarone	Aripiprazole	Atenolol
Calcitonin	Carbamazepine	Chlorpromazine
Clomiphene	Conjugated estrogens	Ferrous sulfate

Thyroid Function Tests (Thyroid-Stimulating Hormone (TSH), Thyrotropin-Releasing Hormone (TRH), Thyroxine-Binding Globulin (TBG), Thyroxine (T4), Free Thyroxine (T4), Free Thyroxine Index (FTI), Triiodothyronine (T3), Free Triiodothyronine (Free T3)

Medications that may increase TSH levels:

Iodine	Levothyroxine	Lithium
Lovastatin	Methimazole	Metoclopramide
Morphine	Phenytoin	Potassium iodine
Prazosin	Prednisone	Propranolol
Radiographic agents	Rifampin	Sumatriptan
Tamoxifen	THR	Valproic acid

Medications that may decrease TSH levels:

Amiodarone	Anabolic steroids	Aspirin
Carbamazepine	Clofibrate	Corticosteroids
Danazol	Dopamine	Fenoldopam
Growth hormone	Heparin	Hydrocortisone
Interferon alfa-2	Levothyroxine	Nifedipine
Octreotide	Peginterferon α-2a	Somatostatin
Steroids	T3	Thyroxine
Troleandomycin		

Thyrotropin-Releasing Hormone (TRH)
Normal Values
Adults: baseline TSH < 10 µ/mL
Stimulated TSH: more than double baseline

Nutritional Significance

TRH test evaluates the responsiveness of the anterior pituitary gland. The patient is given an IV injection of TRH and then the TSH level is measured. In hyperthyroidism, there is either a slight increase or no change in the TSH level because the pituitary production of TSH is suppressed by the circulating levels of T3 and T4. In primary hypothyroidism (thyroid failure), the

THYROID FUNCTION TESTS (THYROID-STIMULATING HORMONE (TSH), THYROTROPIN-RELEASING HORMONE (TRH), THYROXINE-BINDING GLOBULIN (TBG), THYROXINE (T_4), FREE THYROXINE (T_4), FREE THYROXINE INDEX (FTI), TRIIODOTHYRONINE (T_3), FREE TRIIODOTHYRONINE (FREE T_3)

TSH response is 2 to 3 times the normal response. In secondary hypothyroidism (anterior pituitary failure), there is no TSH response. In tertiary hypothyroidism (hypothalamic failure), there is a delayed rise in TSH level. Multiple injections of TRH are needed to stimulate a normal TSH response.

The TRH test is useful to distinguish between primary depression from manic-depressive psychiatric illness and from secondary types of depression. In primary depression, the TRH-induced TSH response is blunted. Patients with other forms of depression have normal TRH-induced TSH responses.

Abnormal TRH with:
- Hypothyroidism
- Psychiatric depression
- Acute starvation
- Hyperthyroidism
- Old age

THYROID FUNCTION TESTS (THYROID-STIMULATING HORMONE (TSH), THYROTROPIN-RELEASING HORMONE (TRH), THYROXINE-BINDING GLOBULIN (TBG), THYROXINE (T4), FREE THYROXINE (T4), FREE THYROXINE INDEX (FTI), TRIIODOTHYRONINE (T3), FREE TRIIODOTHYRONINE (FREE T3)

THYROXINE-BINDING GLOBULIN (TBG)
NORMAL VALUES

Age	Male	Female
1-5 days:	2.2-4.2 mg/dL ; 22-42 mg/L (SI)	2.2-4.2 mg/dL ; 22-42 mg/L (SI)
1-11 mos:	1.6-3.6 mg/dL 16-35 mg/L (SI)	1.7-3.7 mg/dL ; 17-37 mg/L (SI)
1-9 yr:	1.2-2.8 mg/dL ; 12-28mg/L (SI)	1.5-2.7 mg/dL ; 15-275 mg/L (SI)
10-19 yr:	1.4-2.6 mg/dL ; 14-26 mg/L (SI)	1.4-3.0 mg/dL ; 14-30 mg/L (SI)
Adults:	1.7-3.6 mg/dL ; 17-36 mg/L (SI)	1.7-3.6 mg/dL ; 17-36 mg/L (SI)

NUTRITIONAL SIGNIFICANCE

TBG is the major thyroid hormone protein carrier. When TBG is elevated, total T3 and total T4 are also elevated because more T3 and T4 are bound to the carrier protein. Less free, T3 and T4 is available. Low levels of free T3 and T4 stimulate the release of TSH to produce higher levels of T3 and T4.

In some cases only T4 is elevated. More testing is required to determine if the abnormal level is due to high levels of TBG or caused by hyperthyroidism. Thyroid hormone- binding ratio (THBR) can be used to estimate TBG levels. Protein status can affect levels of TBG. Patients with malnutrition may have low TBG related to protein status rather than thyroid disease.

Thyroid Function Tests (Thyroid-Stimulating Hormone (TSH), Thyrotropin-Releasing Hormone (TRH), Thyroxine-Binding Globulin (TBG), Thyroxine (T_4), Free Thyroxine (T_4), Free Thyroxine Index (FTI), Triiodothyronine (T_3), Free Triiodothyronine (Free T_3)

TBG Increased with:
- Pregnancy
- Estrogen replacement therapy
- Estrogen-producing tumors
- Infectious hepatitis
- Genetic increased TBG
- Acute intermittent porphyria
- Hypothyroidism(occasionally)
- Late-stage HIV infections

TBG Decreased with:
- Protein-losing enteropathies
- Testosterone-producing tumors
- Malnutrition
- Protein-losing nephropathy
- Ovarian failure
- Major stress
- Acromegaly
- Chronic liver disease

Medications that may cause increased levels of TBG

Carbamazepine	Clofibrate	Diethylstilbestrol
Erythropoietin	Estrogens	Mestranol
Methadone	Oral contraceptives	Perphenazine
Phenothiazine	Progesterone	Raloxifene
Tamoxifen		

Medications that may cause decreased levels of TBG

Anabolic steroids	Asparaginase	Colestipol
Corticosteroids	Corticotropin	Cortisone
Danazol	Fluoxymesterone	Methyltestosterone
Nandrolone	Norethandrolone	Norethindrone
Oxymetholone	Phenytoin	Prednisone
Propranolol	Stanozolol	

Thyroid Function Tests (Thyroid-Stimulating Hormone (TSH), Thyrotropin-Releasing Hormone (TRH), Thyroxine-Binding Globulin (TBG), Thyroxine (T4), Free Thyroxine (T4), Free Thyroxine Index (FTI), Triiodothyronine (T3), Free Triiodothyronine (Free T3)

Thyroxine (T4)
Normal Values

1-3 days:	11-22 mcg/dL ; 142-283 nmol/L (SI)
1-2 wks:	10-16 mcg/dL ; 129-206 nmol/L (SI)
1-12 mos:	8-16 mcg/dL; 103-206 nmol/L (SI)
1-5 yrs:	7-15 mcg/dL; 90-193 nmol/L (SI)
5-10 yrs:	6-13 mcg/dL ; 77- 167 nmol/L (SI)
10-15 yrs:	5-12 mcg/dL ; 64-154 nmol/L (SI)
Adult females:	5-12 mcg /dL; 64-154 nmol/L (SI)
males:	4-12 mcg /dL; 51-154 nmol/L (SI)
> 60 yrs:	5-11 mcg /dL; 64-142 nmol/L (SI)

Free Thyroxine (T4)

0-4 days:	2-6 ng/dL; 26-77 pmol/L (SI)
2 wks- 20 yr:	0.8-2.0 ng/dL; 10-26 pmol/L (SI)
Adults:	0.8-2.8 ng/dL; 10-36 pmol/L (SI)

Nutritional Significance

The serum thyroxine test measures the total amount of T4 in the blood. Over 99 percent of all T4 is bound to protein and 1-5 percent of total T4 is free or unbound. The free T4 is the metabolically active thyroid hormone. Results for total T4 are affected by TBG levels. As levels of TBG proteins increase, a falsely elevated level of T4 will result. Pregnancy and hormone replacement therapy can increase TGB and cause the T4 to be falsely elevated.

Hypoproteinemia can cause low levels of TGB and subsequently lower levels of total T4. Malnutrition can decrease

Thyroid Function Tests (Thyroid-Stimulating Hormone (TSH), Thyrotropin-Releasing Hormone (TRH), Thyroxine-Binding Globulin (TBG), Thyroxine (T4), Free Thyroxine (T4), Free Thyroxine Index (FTI), Triiodothyronine (T3), Free Triiodothyronine (Free T3)

TGB and cause total T4 to be falsely depressed. Low levels suggest hypothyroidism. Newborns are screened for T4 to detect hypothyroidism and if needed begin treatment to prevent mental retardation.

Increased with:
- Primary hyperthyroid states:
  - Graves' disease
  - Plummer's disease
  - toxic thyroid adenoma
- Acute thyroiditis
- Hashimoto's thyroiditis
- Factitious hyperthyroidism
- Struma ovarii
- Hepatitis
- Congenital hyperproteinemia

Decreased with:
- Hypothyroid states:
  - cretinism
  - surgical ablation
  - myxedema
- Pituitary insufficiency
- Hypothalamic failure
- Iodine deficiency
- Non-thyroid diseases:
  - renal failure
  - Cushing's Syndrome
  - advanced cancers
  - cirrhosis
  - surgery
  - protein depleted states

Medications that may increase free T4 levels:

Amiodarone	Aspirin	Carbamazepine
Danazol	Enoxaparin	Erythropoietin
Furosemide	Levothyroxine	Phenytoin
Propranolol	Propylthiouracil	Radiographic agents
Tamoxifen	Thyroxine	Valproic acid

Thyroid Function Tests (Thyroid-Stimulating Hormone (TSH), Thyrotropin-Releasing Hormone (TRH), Thyroxine-Binding Globulin (TBG), Thyroxine (T4), Free Thyroxine (T4), Free Thyroxine Index (FTI), Triiodothyronine (T3), Free Triiodothyronine (Free T3)

Medications that may decrease free T4 levels:

Amiodarone	Anabolic steroids	Carbamazepine
Clofibrate	Corticosteroids	Conjugated estrogens
Isotretinoin	Levothyroxine	Lithium
Mestranol	Methadone	Methimazole
Norethindrone	Octreotide	Oral contraceptives
Oxacillin	Phenobarbital	Phenytoin
Ranitidine		

Free Thyroxine Index (FTI)
Normal Values
Adults: 0.8-2.4 ng/dL; 10-31 pmol/L (SI)
Adult index: 1.5-4.5 (if units are eliminated)

Nutritional Significance

FTI measures the amount of free T4 and is not affected by thyroid-binding globulin abnormalities. This index is useful in diagnosing hyperthyroidism and hypothyroidism in patients with abnormal TGB levels as a result of certain medications.

FTI Increased with:
- Graves' disease
- Plummer's disease
- Toxic thyroiditis
- Factitious hyperthyroidism
- Struma ovarii
- Hyperthyroidism
- Acute thyroiditis

FTI Decreased with:
- Hypothyroidism
- Cretinism
- Surgical ablation
- Myxedema
- Pituitary insufficiency
- Hypothalamic failure
- Iodine deficiency

Thyroid Function Tests (Thyroid-Stimulating Hormone (TSH), Thyrotropin-Releasing Hormone (TRH), Thyroxine-Binding Globulin (TBG), Thyroxine (T4), Free Thyroxine (T4), Free Thyroxine Index (FTI), Triiodothyronine (T3), Free Triiodothyronine (Free T3)

Medications that may increase FTI levels:

Amiodarone	Aspirin	Carbamazepine
Danazol	Enoxaparin	Erythropoietin
Furosemide	Levothyroxine	Phenytoin
Propranolol	Propylthiouracil	Radiographic agents
Tamoxifen	Thyroxine	Valproic acid

Medications that may decrease FTI levels:

Amiodarone	Anabolic steroids	Carbamazepine
Clofibrate	Corticosteroids	Conjugated estrogens
Isotretinoin	Levothyroxine	Lithium
Mestranol	Methadone	Methimazole
Norethindrone	Octreotide	Oral contraceptives
Oxacillin	Phenobarbital	Phenytoin
Ranitidine		

Triiodothyronine (T3)
Normal Values

1-3 days:	100-740 ng/dL; 1.5-11.4 nmol/L (SI)
1-11 mos:	105-245 ng/dL; 1.6-3.8 nmol/L (SI)
1-5 yrs:	105-270 ng/dL; 1.6-4.1 nmol/L (SI)
6-10 yrs:	95-240 ng/dL; 1.5-3.7 nmol/L (SI)
11-15 yrs	80-215 ng/dL; 1.2-3.3 nmol/L (SI)
16-20 yrs:	80-210 ng/dL; 1.2-3.2 nmol/L (SI)
20-50 yrs:	70-205 ng/dL; 1.1-3.1 nmol/L (SI)
> 50 yrs:	40-180 ng/dL; 0.6-2.8 nmol/L (SI)

Free Triiodothyronine (FT3)
Normal Values

Adults:	260-480 pg/dL; 4.0-7.4 pmol/L (SI)

THYROID FUNCTION TESTS (THYROID-STIMULATING HORMONE (TSH), THYROTROPIN-RELEASING HORMONE (TRH), THYROXINE-BINDING GLOBULIN (TBG), THYROXINE (T4), FREE THYROXINE (T4), FREE THYROXINE INDEX (FTI), TRIIODOTHYRONINE (T3), FREE TRIIODOTHYRONINE (FREE T3)

NUTRITIONAL SIGNIFICANCE

Triiodothyronine is formed when one diiodotyrosine combines with a monoiodothyronine. The majority of T3 is formed in the liver via conversion of T4 to T3. About 7-10 percent of thyroid hormone is composed of T3. About 70 percent of the T3 is bound to either thyroxine-binding protein or albumin. Hypothyroidism is suspected when T3 is below normal ranges. If the patient has severe non-thyroid diseases, the levels of T3 can be diminished because the liver is unable to convert T4 to T3. Very small quantities are unbound or 'free'. It is the 'free' T3 that is metabolically active. Free T3 is not impacted by changes in serum proteins, like total T3. The purpose of doing a FT3 is to rule out toxicosis, evaluate for thyroid replacement therapy and to clarify protein-binding abnormalities. Hyperthyroidism is associated with elevated levels of T3 and T4. If T3 is elevated and T4 is normal, T3 toxicosis is suspected.

FT3 Increased with:
- Graves' disease
- Pregnancy (↑TBG)
- Hepatitis (↑TBG)
- Congenital hyperproteinemia (↑TBG)
- Toxic thyroid adenoma
- Plummer's disease
- Acute thyroiditis

FT3 Decreased with:
- Cretinism
- Surgical removal of thyroid
- Myxedema
- Pituitary insufficiency
- Hypothalamic failure
- Protein wasting diseases
- Malnutrition
- Iodine deficiency

THYROID FUNCTION TESTS (THYROID-STIMULATING HORMONE (TSH), THYROTROPIN-RELEASING HORMONE (TRH), THYROXINE-BINDING GLOBULIN (TBG), THYROXINE (T4), FREE THYROXINE (T4), FREE THYROXINE INDEX (FTI), TRIIODOTHYRONINE (T3), FREE TRIIODOTHYRONINE (FREE T3)

FT3 Increased with:
- Factitious hyperthyroidism
- Struma ovarii

FT3 Decreased with:
- Renal failure
- Hepatic disease/cirrhosis
- Cushing's syndrome
- Surgery
- Advanced cancers

Medications that may increase T3 or FT3 levels:
Amiodarone	Amphetamine	Clofibrate
Erythropoietin	Estropipate	Fluorouracil
Insulin	Levothyroxine	Mestranol
Methadone	Opiates	Oral contraceptives
Phenothiazine	Phenytoin	Propylthiouracil
Ranitidine	Tamoxifen	Terbutaline
Thyrotropin-releasing hormones		Valproic acid

Medications that may decrease T3 or FT3 levels:
Amiodarone	Anabolic steroids	Asparaginase
Aspirin	Atenolol	Carbamazepine
Cholestyramine	Cimetidine	Clomiphene
Clomipramine	Cotrimoxazole	Corticosteroids
Danazol	Dexamethasone	Diclofenac
Furosemide	Glucocorticoids	Hydrocortisone
Interferon alfa-2	Iodine	Isotretinoin
Lithium	Methimazole	Metoprolol
Mitotane	Naproxen	Netilmicin
Oral contraceptives	Penicillamine	Phenobarbital
Phenytoin	Potassium iodine	Prednisone
Propranolol	Propylthiouracil	Radiographic agents
Reserpine	Salsalate	Somatostatin
Stanozolol	Sulfonylureas	Theophylline

TRIGLYCERIDES

NORMAL VALUES

Age	Male	Female
1-9 yrs	30-100 mg/dL; 0.34-1.13 mmol/L (SI)	35-110 mg/dL; 0.4-1.24 mmol/L (SI)
10-14 yrs	32-125 mg/dL; 0.36-1.41 mmol/L (SI)	37-131 mg/dL; 0.42-1.48 mmol/L (SI)
15-20 yrs	37-148 mg/dL; 0.42-1.67 mmol/L (SI)	39-124 mg/dL; .44-1.4 mmol/L (SI)
20-24 yrs	34-137 mg/dL; 0.38-1.55 mmol/L (SI)	32-100 mg/dL; 0.36-1.13 mmol/L (SI)
Adults	40-150 mg/dL; 0.45-1.70 mmol/L	35-135 mg/dL; 0.40-1.52 mmol/L (SI)

NUTRITIONAL SIGNIFICANCE

Triglycerides are a form of fat found in the bloodstream. They are transported in the blood by VLDL and LDL). The liver synthesizes triglycerides, which are composed of carbon, hydrogen and oxygen (glycerol) and three fatty acids. Their role is to store energy. When blood levels exceed norms the triglycerides are deposited into the fatty tissues. Excess levels of triglycerides are seen in individuals consuming a high fat diet and high levels of alcohol. Individuals with hyperthyroidism will have reduced levels because of an increased catabolism of VLDL, the main triglyceride carrying lipoprotein. Recent studies have demonstrated that children who have elevated triglyceride levels are at significant risk of cardiovascular disease as are adults. Obesity, diabetes and inactivity increase the risk of cardiovascular disease significantly.

Patients need to fast for 12-14 hours prior to the test.

TRIGLYCERIDES

RELATED TESTS: cholesterol, lipoproteins

Increased with:
- Glycogen storage disease
- Hyperlipidemias
- Hypertension
- Myocardial infarction
- Hypothyroidism
- High carbohydrate diet
- High fat diet
- Poorly controlled diabetes
- Nephrotic syndrome
- Alcoholic cirrhosis
- Pregnancy
- Pancreatitis
- Gout
- Werner's syndrome
- Downs syndrome
- Anorexia nervosa

Decreased with:
- Malabsorption
- Malnutrition
- Hyperthyroidism
- AIDS
- COPD
- Brain infarction

Medications that may increase levels:

Abarelix	Acetylsalicylic acid	Amiodarone
Ardeparin	Ascorbic acid	Atenolol
Beta blockers	Bisoprolol	Carbamazepine
Carvedilol	Casodex	Chlordane
Chlorothiazide	Chlorthalidone	Cholestyramine
Colchicine	Cyclosporine	Danazol
Didanosine	Enalapril	Enfuvirtide
Estrogen/progestin	Estrogens	Etretinate
Fluconazole	Fluvastatin	Fosamprenavir
Furosemide	Glucocorticoids	Glycerin
Goserelin	Hydrochlorothiazide	Interferon alfa-2a
Isotretinoin	Itraconazole	Labetalol
Levothyroxine	Methyclothiazide	Methyldopa
Metoprolol	Miconazole	Mirtazapine
Nadolol	Nafarelin	Nandrolone
Norfloxacin	Ofloxacin	Olmesartan
Oral contraceptives	Perindopril	Pindolol
Polythiazide	Prazosin	Prednisolone
Propranolol	Radioactive iodine	Risperidone

TRIGLYCERIDES

Medications that may increase levels:
Ritonavir
Spironolactone
Thiazides
Tretinoin
Zalcitabine
Simvastatin
Tamoxifen
Ticlopidine
Trichlormethiazide
Sotalol
Tenofovir
Timolol
Warfarin

Medications that may decrease levels:
Acarbose
Amiodarone
Ascorbic acid
Azathioprine
Carvedilol
Chlorthalidone
Colestipol
Diltiazem
Estrogens
Fluvastatin
HMG CoA-reductase inhibitors
Indomethacin
Levodopa
LMP heparin
Metformin
Nicardipine
Nisoldipine
Pentoxifylline
Prazosin
Psyllium
Terazosin
Verapamil
ACE inhibitors
Amlodipine
Asparaginase
Bisoprolol
Cerivastatin
Cholestyramine
Danazol
Doxazosin
Fenofibrate
Gemfibrozil
Hydroxychloroquine

Insulin
Levonorgestrel
Lovastatin
Methimazole
Nicotinic acid
Norethindrone
Pindolol
Prednisolone
Simvastatin
Troglitazone
Acetylsalicylic acid
Anabolic steroids
Atorvastatin
Captopril
Chenodiol
Clofibrate
Dexfenfluramine
Enalapril
Flaxseed oil
Glyburide
Hydroxyurea

Ketoconazole
Levothyroxine
Medroxyprogesterone
Niacin
Nifedipine
Oxandrolone
Pravastatin
Probucol
Stanozolol
Unfractionated heparin

TROPONIN (CARDIAC-SPECIFIC TROPONIN [cTnT], CARDIAC-SPECIFIC I [cTnI])

NORMAL VALUES
Cardiac troponin T   < 0.2 ng/mL
Cardiac troponin I :   < 0.3 ng/mL

NUTRITIONAL SIGNIFICANCE

Cardiac-specific troponin test is used to evaluate patients complaining of chest pain with suspected acute coronary ischemic syndromes. They are also used to predict the risk of future cardiac events. Troponins are proteins found in skeletal and cardiac muscle. They are involved in the regulation of myosin and actin. There are two cardiac-specific troponin: cardiac troponin T (cTnT) and cardiac troponin I (cTnI), which become elevated about 3 hours after a myocardial injury. Levels of cTnI remain elevated for 7 to 10 days after a myocardial infarction and cTnT are elevated for up to 14 days. Cardiac-specific troponins are not affected by skeletal muscle injury.

Cardiac troponins are preferred to measuring LDH or CK-MB enzymes. They are almost always normal in noncardiac muscle diseases. If the patient has reinfarction, the cardiac-specific tests are not useful because they could be elevated from the first ischemic event. Troponin T levels are falsely elevated in dialysis patients.

RELATED TESTS: CK-MB, myoglobin, ECG

Cardiac-related Increases:
- Myocardial injury in surgery
- Myocardial infarction
- Myocarditis

Non-Cardiac Increases:
- Chronic renal failure
- Acute muscle trauma
- Rhabdomyolysis

VITAMIN A, RETINOL

NORMAL VALUES
Adults: 20-80 mcg/dL ; 0.7-2.8 µmol/L(SI)
CRITICAL VALUES < 10 mcg/dL; 0.35 µmol/L(SI)

NUTRITIONAL SIGNIFICANCE

Vitamin A (retinol) is a fat soluble vitamin required for the formation of rhodopsin, a photoreceptor pigment in the retina. It also helps maintain epithelial tissues. Normally, the liver stores 80 to 90 percent of the body's vitamin A. To use vitamin A, the body releases it into the circulation bound to prealbumin and retinol-binding protein. β-Carotene and other provitamin carotenoids, contained in green leafy and yellow vegetables and deep- or bright-colored fruits, are converted to vitamin A.

Vitamin A requirements are expressed as retinol activity equivalents (RAE) because provitamin A carotenoids have less vitamin A activity than preformed vitamin A. 12 micrograms β-carotene = 1 RAE and 1 mcg retinol= 1 RAE.

Primary vitamin A deficiency can result from inadequate intake, fat malabsorption, or liver disorders. Deficiency impairs immunity and hematopoiesis and causes skin rashes and xerophthalmia (night blindness). Xerophthalmia, due to primary deficiency, is a common cause of blindness among young children in developing countries.

Secondary vitamin A deficiency may be due to decreased bioavailability of provitamin A carotenoids or to interference with

VITAMIN A, RETINOL

absorption, storage, or transport of vitamin A. Interference with absorption or storage is likely in sprue, cystic fibrosis, pancreatic insufficiency, duodenal bypass, chronic diarrhea, cirrhosis, bile duct obstruction and giardiasis. Vitamin A deficiency is common in prolonged malnutrition not only because the diet is deficient but also because vitamin A storage and transport is defective.

Deficiency symptoms include impaired dark adaptation of the eyes. If untreated, xerophthalmia results from keratinization of the eyes. There is xerosis of eye and thickening of the conjunctivae and corneas. Superficial foamy patches composed of epithelial debris and secretions on the exposed bulbar conjunctiva (Bitot's spots) develop. In advanced deficiency, the cornea becomes hazy and can develop keratomalacia. Keratinization of the skin and of the mucous membranes in the respiratory, GI, and urinary tracts can occur. Drying, scaling, and follicular thickening of the skin and respiratory infections can result. Immunity is generally impaired.

In young children, growth retardation and infections are common among children. Mortality rate can exceed 50 percent in children with severe vitamin A deficiency.

Vitamin A toxicity can be acute or chronic. Plasma retinol levels increase from normal ranges to over 100 mcg/dL; 3.49 µmol/L. Symptoms include changes in hair, alopecia of the eyebrows, dry, rough skin, dry eyes, and cracked lips. Later, severe headache, pseudotumor cerebri, and generalized weakness

VITAMIN A, RETINOL

develop. Cortical hyperostosis of bone, hepatomegaly, arthralgia, splenomegaly and fractures may occur.

RELATED TESTS: RBP, PAB

Increased with:
- Supplemental Vitamin A
- Supplemental β-carotene

Decreased with:
- Malnutrition
- Malabsorption syndromes
- Sprue
- Cystic fibrosis
- Pancreatic insufficiency
- RNY gastric bypass
- Duodenal bypass
- Chronic diarrhea
- Bile duct obstruction
- Giardiasis
- Cirrhosis
- AIDS

VITAMIN B6

NORMAL VALUES
Adults: 5-24 ng/mL; 30-144 nmol/L (SI)

NUTRITIONAL SIGNIFICANCE

Vitamin B6 includes pyridoxine, pyridoxal, and pyridoxamine, which are metabolized to pyridoxal phosphate (PLP). PLP acts as a coenzyme for numerous enzymes involved in the metabolism of amino acids, neurotransmitters (serotonin, epinephrine, norepinephrine, γ-aminobutyric acid), and porphyrin precursors of heme and steroids. It is required for the conversion of tryptophan to niacin, the release of glucose from glycogen, the biosynthesis of sphingolipids to myelin sheaths of nerve cells and the conversion of folate into its active form. Vitamin B6 is present in most foods and is absorbed by passive diffusion in the jejunum and ileum.

While a dietary deficiency is rare, secondary deficiency may result from malnutrition, malabsorption, alcoholism, or use of pyridoxine-inactivating medications. Deficiency symptoms can include weakness, sleepiness, cheilosis, glossitis, stomatitis, anemia, peripheral neuropathy, a pellagra-like syndrome, depression, confusion, EEG abnormalities, anemia, impaired cell-mediated immunity and seizures.

The toxic effect of long-term, excessive pyridoxine consumption initially presents as bilateral numbness and tingling in the feet and legs. Pyridoxine inhibits methionine metabolism, causing an increase in S-adenosylmethionine, which in turn

Vitamin B6

inhibits myelin synthesis. In general, exposure of 2 g/d is needed to cause the neuropathy, but cases due to longstanding use of as little as 200 mg/d have been reported. Recovery is usually good after pyridoxine is stopped. This is the only water soluble vitamin to cause a neuropathy when taken to excess.

Related Tests: folic acid, vitamin B12, CBC, homocysteine

Increased with:
- Supplemental B6

Decreased with:
- Malnutrition
- Malabsorption syndromes
- Alcoholism
- Sickle cell anemia

Medications that may decrease levels:

Cycloserine	Estradiol	Ethinyl
Hydralazine	Isoniazid	Mestranol
Penicillamine		

VITAMIN B12

NORMAL VALUES

Adults: 160-950 pg/mL; 118-701 pmol/L (SI)

NUTRITIONAL SIGNIFICANCE

Vitamin B12 is required for the conversion of methyltetrahydrofolate to the active form of folic acid. This reaction is essential for the synthesis of nucleic acids and amino acids and for the normal formation and function of RBC. When B12 is deficient in the diet or underutilized due to a lack of intrinsic factor (IF), the formation and function of RBC is impacted. In a B12 deficiency or folic acid deficiency the RBC are large and immature. Theses abnormal RBC cannot conform to the size of small capillaries. Instead, they fracture and hemolyze, thus shortening their lifespan. Pernicious anemia occurs.

Vitamin B12 is found in animal products and B12 fortified foods. The gastric acid in the stomach breaks B12 from its binding proteins. B12 requires IF, secreted from the parietal cells in the stomach, for absorption in the distal ileum.

A deficiency of B12, or pernicious anemia is due to:
- Deficiency of IF
- Lack of gastric acid to separate vitamin B12 from its binding proteins
- Malabsorption of vitamin B12 due to disease of the small terminal ileum, IBS or neoplasm

Symptoms of pernicious anemia include symmetric glove-and-stocking paresthesias, or tingling in the distal aspect of the toes,

VITAMIN B12

numbness, coldness, a pins-and-needles feeling, and weakness, lightheadedness, vertigo, tinnitus, palpitations, angina, heart failure, cardiomegaly, pallor, tachycardia, and hepatosplenomegaly. GI symptoms include a sore, beefy red tongue and anorexia. Macrocytic anemia is seen in about 60% of cases.

In late stages, manifestations include moderate muscular wasting, optic atrophy, sphincter dysfunction, and mental disturbances such as mild dementia (which is often the first symptom and clinically indistinguishable from other dementias), disorientation, depression, psychosis, and persecutory delusions.

RELATED TESTS: folic acid, Schilling test, CBC, MMA

Increased with:
- Leukemia
- Polycythemia vera
- Severe liver dysfunction
- Myeloproliferative disease

Decreased with:
- Pernicious anemia
- Malabsorption syndromes
- Inflammatory bowel disease
- Resection of terminal ileum
- Atrophic gastritis
- Zollinger-Ellison syndrome
- Large proximal gastrectomy
- Achlorhydria
- Pregnancy
- Ascorbic acid deficiency
- Folate deficiency
- Intestinal worm infestation
- Alcoholism
- Liver disease
- Bariatric procedures

Medications that may increase levels:
Chloral hydrate   Omeprazole

Vitamin B12

Medications that may decrease levels:

Alcohol	Aminoglycosides	Aminosalicylic acid
Anticonvulsants	Ascorbic acid	Chlorpromazine
Cholestyramine	Colchicine	Metformin
Neomycin	Octreotide	Oral contraceptives
Ranitidine	Rifampin	

VITAMIN D, 25(OH)D

NORMAL VALUES (varies by organization)

Organization	Deficiency	Insufficiency	Sufficiency
WHO, 2008	< 20 ng/mL; < 50 nmol/L	20-31 ng/mL; 50-80 nmol/L	> 32 ng/mL; >80 nmol/L
IOF(2010)	No cutpoint	No cutpoint	> 30 ng/mL; >75 nmol/L
IOM(2011)	<12 ng/mL; <30 nmol/L	No cutpoint	> 12 ng/mL; >30 nmol/L

CRITICAL VALUE   < 8 ng/mL; < 20 nmol/L (SI)

NUTRITIONAL SIGNIFICANCE

Vitamin D is a group of fat-soluble sterols naturally found in a few foods. The primary source of vitamin D is from sunlight (UVB rays). The physiologically important forms of vitamin D are vitamin D2 or ergocalciferol and D3 cholecalciferol. These serve as precursors for the active form of vitamin D, 1,25 (OH2D3). The conversion to the active form is regulated by parathyroid hormone (PTH) and serum concentrations of calcium and phosphate.

Vitamin D serves many roles in the body including bone health, immunogenic and antitumor activity, risk reduction of many chronic and autoimmune diseases. Inadequate intakes of vitamin D and inadequate exposure to sunlight can result in a vitamin D deficiency causing rickets in children and osteomalacia in adults. Vitamin D deficiency causes hypocalcemia which stimulates production of PTH causing hyperparathyroidism. Hyperparathyroidism increases absorption, bone mobilization, and renal conservation of calcium but increases excretion of phosphate. As a result, the serum level of calcium may be normal,

Vitamin D 25(OH)D

but because of hypophosphatemia, bone mineralization is impaired. Secondary vitamin D deficiency may be due to chronic renal failure, severe liver disease and gastrointestinal losses from malabsorption syndromes or bariatric procedures. Individuals with dark skin pigmentation, those wearing full body clothing and who live far from the equator are at greater risk of developing a deficiency.

Symptoms of a vitamin D deficiency in adults include muscle aches and weakness, bone pain and minimal trauma fractures. In young infants, rickets causes a softening of the skull. In older infants and children with rickets, sitting, crawling and walking can be delayed. Deformities such as bowlegs and knock-knees may develop in untreated children.

Related Tests: ALP, PTH, urinary Ca, serum Ca, PO4

Increased with:
- Supplemental Vitamin D
- Exposure to UVB rays

Decreased with:
- Severe liver dysfunction
- Malabsorption syndromes
- Inflammatory bowel disease
- Chronic renal failure
- Bariatric procedures
- Hypoparathyroidism
- Nephrotic syndrome
- Peritoneal syndrome
- Celiac disease & sprue
- Cystic fibrosis
- Pancreatic insufficiency
- Chronic steatorrhea
- Hereditary vitamin D dependent rickets

Medications that may decrease levels:

Carbamazepine	Isoniazid	Phenobarbital
Phenytoin	Rifampin	Theophylline

VITAMIN E

NORMAL VALUES
Adults: 5-20 mcg/L ; 11.6-46 µmol/L (SI)

CRITICAL VALUES
α-tocopherol < 5 mcg/L ; < 11.6 µmol/L (SI)
α-tocopherol to total plasma lipids < 0.8 mg/g total lipids

NUTRITIONAL SIGNIFICANCE

Vitamin E is a group of compounds including tocopherols and tocotrienols that have similar biologic activities. The most biologically active is α-tocopherol. These compounds act as antioxidants that prevent lipid peroxidation of polyunsaturated fatty acids in cellular membranes. Plasma tocopherol levels vary with total plasma lipid levels.

Vitamin E deficiency is uncommon in healthy adults eating a variety of foods. It can occur in adults with fat malabsorption syndromes including Crohn's disease, cystic fibrosis, short bowel syndrome and bariatric procedures. The main symptoms are hemolytic anemia and neurologic deficits. Diagnosis is based on either plasma levels of vitamin E or measuring the ratio of plasma α-tocopherol to total plasma lipids. Abnormal plasma lipid levels can affect vitamin E status. A low ratio suggests a vitamin E deficiency. Measuring RBC hemolysis in response to peroxide can suggest a vitamin E deficiency, but this test is nonspecific. Hemolysis increases as vitamin E deficiency impairs RBC stability.

Vitamin E toxicity is rare even in adults who take relatively large amounts for months to years. The most significant risk is

VITAMIN E

increased bleeding times. Occasionally muscle weakness, fatigue, nausea and diarrhea may occur.

RELATED TESTS: CBC, lipid profile

Increased with:
- Supplemental vitamin E

Decreased with:
- Inadequate dietary intake
- Malabsorption syndromes
- Bariatric procedures
- Abetalipoproteinemia
- Cholestatic hepatobiliary disease
- Pancreatitis
- Short bowel syndrome
- Cystic fibrosis

WHITE BLOOD CELL (WBC) COUNT & DIFFERENTIAL COUNT

NORMAL VALUES TOTAL WBC
Newborn	9000-30,000/mm³ ; 9-30.0 X 10^9 /L (SI)
Child under 2 yr	6200-17,000/mm³; 6.2-17.0 X 10^9 /L (SI)
Adults/children >2 yr:	5000-10,000/mm³; 5-10.0 X 10^9 /L (SI)

DIFFERENTIAL COUNT	%	ABSOLUTE (per mm³)
Neutrophils	55% to 70%	2500-8000
Lymphocytes	20% to 40%	1000-4000
Monocytes	2% to 8%	100-700
Eosinophils	1% to 4%	50-500
Basophils	0.5% to 1.0 %	25-100

Total Lymphocyte Count (TLC) is derived using WBC and the differential:

$$TLC = WBC \times \frac{\% \text{ Lymphocytes}}{100} \text{ (in differential)}$$

NUTRITIONAL SIGNIFICANCE

WBC fight infection and react to foreign bodies or tissues. They are divided into two types: granulocytes and agranulocytes. The granulocytes have granules in their cytoplasm and include neutrophils, basophils, and eosinophils. Granulocytes have multilobed nuclei and are sometimes called polymorphonuclear leukocytes or PMN or 'polys.' The agranulocytes include lymphocytes and monocytes. They have no granules in the cytoplasm and have a small single nuclei.

The WBC count has two components;
1) total number of leukocytes in 1mm³ of peripheral venus blood
2) differential count or the percentage of each type of leukocyte present.

White Blood Cell (WBC) Count & Differential Count

The differential count is based on a total of 100 percent of the leukocytes. When one type increases there is an automatic decrease in the percentage of another type. Neutrophils and lymphocytes make up the bulk of the differential (75-90 percent). Other types include monocytes, eosinophils and basophils.

An increase in total WBC or leukocytes usually suggests infection, inflammation, tissue necrosis or leukemic neoplasia. Trauma and stress, whether it be physical or emotional, may induce leukocytosis (increase in WBC count). Individuals who have had a splenectomy will have a persistent mild to moderate elevation of WBC counts. Elderly patients may not experience an elevated WBC count with an infection. Critical values are greater than 30,000/ mm^3; 30.0 X 10^9 /L (SI).

Leukopenia or a decrease in WBC count may suggest bone marrow failure following antineoplastic chemotherapy, radiation therapy, bone marrow infiltrative diseases, overwhelming infections, dietary deficiencies and autoimmune diseases. Critical values:

- impaired immunity <1800 > 900 mm^3;< 1.8 > 0.9 X 10^9 /L (SI)
- anergy or no immunity < 900 mm^3; <0.9 X 10^9 /L (SI)

Neutrophils

Changes in the differential count suggest a variety of conditions. Neutrophils are produced in 7 to 14 days and have a life span of only 6 hours. Phagocytosis is their primary function.

White Blood Cell (WBC) Count & Differential Count

Acute bacterial infections and trauma stimulate neutrophil production resulting in an increased WBC count. When the demand for neutrophils increases there is an increase in immature forms of neutrophils. These are called band or stab cells. An increase in band or stab cells is referred to as a "shift to the left" in WBC production. In other words, there is an ongoing acute bacterial infection and the body has increased its neutrophil production to meet or try to meet the need. However, when a dramatic decrease in neutrophils is seen following a "shift to the left" this does not necessarily mean the patient has improved. For example, it may follow chemotherapy. Medications are used to increase the WBC prior to resuming chemotherapy treatments. However, in cases of overwhelming infections a dramatic decrease in WBC may suggest a "degenerative shift" or bone marrow failure. In other words, the body is losing its ability to produce neutrophils at the rate needed. When the body is unable to produce neutrophils to fight an infection and the supply is depleted, death will occur shortly.

Lymphocytes

Lymphocytes fight chronic bacterial infections and acute viral infections. They are either T-cells or B-cells. The differential count does not separate the T- and B-cells. The lymphocyte percentage represents a total of T-and B-cells. T-cells are primarily involved with cellular-type immune reactions i.e. fungal and viral infections and transplant rejection. The T-cell

White Blood Cell (WBC) Count & Differential Count

secretions stimulate the B-cell response. B-cells participate in antibody production or humoral immunity. When the humoral immunity is activated the B-cells specific to the antigen differentiate into plasma or memory cells. These cells synthesize and release antibodies or immunoglobulins. The antibody binds to the antigen and inactivates it.

Monocytes

The monocytes are also phagocytic cells similar to the neutrophils. They are capable of fighting bacteria. Monocytes are produced more rapidly and have a longer life span. These cells secrete cytokines that regulate the immune response.

Basophils & Eosinophils

Basophils and eosinophils are involved in allergic reactions. For example, when a patient has persistent symptoms of a respiratory infection and antibiotics are ineffective, an increase in eosinophils and a decrease in basophils may indicate an allergic reaction. Parasitic infestations are capable of stimulating these cells. Basophils and eosinophils are phagocytic cells, but do not respond to bacterial or viral infections.

Increased WBC count (leukocytosis):
- Infection
- Leukemic neoplasia
- Trauma
- Stress
- Malignant neoplasms

Decreased WBC Count (leukopenia)
- Drug toxicity (e.g. chloramphenicol)
- Overwhelming infections
- AIDS
- Autoimmune disease

WHITE BLOOD CELL (WBC) COUNT & DIFFERENTIAL COUNT

Increased WBC count (leukocytosis):
- Tissue necrosis
- Inflammation

Decreased WBC Count (leukopenia):
- Dietary deficiency (B_{12} or Fe)
- Bone marrow infiltration myelofibrosis
- Hypersplenism
- Congenital disorders
- Kostmann's syndrome
- Reticular agenesis
- Cartilage-hair hypoplasia
- Shwachman-Diamond syndrome
- Chediak-Higashi syndrome

Medications that may increase levels:

Adrenalin	Allopurinol	Aspirin
Chloroform	Epinephrine	Heparin
Quinine	Steroids	Triamterene

Medications that may decrease levels:

Antibiotics	Anticonvulsants	Antihistamines
Antimetabolites	Antithyroid	Arsenicals
Barbiturates	Chemotherapeutic agents	Diuretics
Sulfonamides		

Etiology of Abnormal WBC Counts for Neutrophils

Elevated: Neutrophilia
- Physical or emotional stress
- Acute suppurative infection
- Myelocytic leukemia
- Trauma
- Cushing's syndrome
- Inflammatory disorders:
  - rheumatic fever
  - thyroiditis
  - rheumatoid arthritis

Decreased: Neutropenia
- Aplastic anemia
- Dietary deficiency
- Overwhelming bacterial & viral infections
  - hepatitis
  - influenza
  - measles
- Radiation therapy
- Addison's disease

White Blood Cell (WBC) Count & Differential Count

Etiology of Abnormal WBC Counts for Neutrophils

Elevated: Neutrophilia
- Metabolic disorders:
  - eclampsia
  - ketoacidosis
  - gout

Decreased: Neutropenia
- Drug toxicity (chemotherapy)

Etiology of Abnormal WBC Counts for Lymphocytes

Elevated: Lymphocytosis
- Chronic bacterial infection
- Viral infection:
  - mumps
  - rubella
- Lymphocytic leukemia
- Multiple myeloma
- Infectious mononucleosis
- Radiation
- Infectious hepatitis

Decreased: Lymphocytopenia
- Leukemia
- Sepsis
- Immunodeficiency diseases
- Systemic lupus erythematosus
- Advanced stages AIDS
- Radiation therapy
- Medications:
  - adrenocorticosteroid
  - antineoplastics

Etiology of Abnormal WBC Counts for Monocytes

Elevated: Monocytosis
- Parasites
- Viral infections
- Tuberculosis
- Chronic ulcerative colitis
- Chronic inflammatory disorders

Decreased: Monocytopenia
- Aplastic anemia
- Hairy-cell leukemia
- Medications:
  - prednisone

Etiology of Abnormal WBC Counts for Basophils

Elevated: Basophilia
- Myeloproliferative disease
- Leukemia
- Uremia

Decreased: Basopenia
- Acute allergic reactions
- Hyperthyroidism
- Stress response

White Blood Cell (WBC) Count & Differential Count

Etiology of Abnormal WBC Counts for Eosinophils

Elevated: Eosinophilia
- Parasitic infections
- Allergic reactions
- Eczema
- Leukemia
- Autoimmune diseases

Decreased: Eosinopenia
- ↑ adrenosteroid production

Zinc (Zn), Plasma

NORMAL VALUES, SERUM
Child 0-10 yrs   0.60-1.2 mcg/mL
Adults (11 yrs +)   0.66-1.1 mcg/mL

CRITICAL VALUE   < 0.6 mcg/mL

NUTRITIONAL SIGNIFICANCE

Zinc is a component of hundreds of enzymes including nicotinamide adenine dinucleotide (NADH) dehydrogenases, RNA and DNA polymerases, and DNA transcription factors as well as alkaline phosphatase, superoxide dismutase, and carbonic anhydrase. Healthy adults eating a variety of foods rarely develop a zinc deficiency. However, a secondary zinc deficiency can occur in some patients with hepatic insufficiency because they lose the ability to retain zinc, in the elderly due to inadequate dietary intakes and in individuals with draining wounds and metabolic stress from sepsis, burns or injury. Also individuals with diabetes mellitus, sickle cell disease chronic renal failure, malabsorption syndromes including weight loss surgery are at risk for a secondary zinc deficiency.

Maternal zinc deficiency can cause fetal malformations and low birth weight. Zinc deficiency in children causes impaired growth hypogeusia and delayed sexual maturation. Symptoms of a zinc deficiency in children and adults includes hypogonadism, alopecia, impaired immunity, anorexia, dermatitis, night blindness, anemia, lethargy and impaired wound healing.

ZINC (ZN), PLASMA

Zinc deficiency is difficult to quantify since many of the symptoms are nonspecific and blood tests are not always available or reliable. Low albumin is common in zinc deficiency since albumin is the primary binding protein for zinc. However, albumin, a negative acute phase protein, is affected by inflammation and many other factors as well. Zinc deficiency diagnosis usually requires a combination of low levels of plasma zinc and increased urinary zinc excretion.

RELATED TESTS: serum iron, TIBC, ferritin, hemoglobin, hematocrit, PAB

Increased with:
- Supplemental zinc

Decreased with:
- Inadequate dietary intake
- High fiber diet
- High phytate diet
- Hepatic cirrhosis
- Ulcerative colitis
- Crohn's disease
- Regional enteritis
- Sprue
- Bariatric procedures
- Neoplastic disease
- Malnutrition
- Burn patients

Medications that may decrease levels:

Anabolic steroids

REFERENCES

Acchiardo SR, Moore LW, Latour, BA (1983) Malnutrition as the main factor in morbidity and mortality of hemodialysis patients. *Kidney Int,* 24:5 - 199 - S203.

Adcock, BB, McKnight, JT (2003) Cobalamin pseudodeficiency due to transcobalamin I deficiency. *South Med J* 95(9):1060—1062.

Ahluwalia N, Lammi-Keef CJ, Bendel RB, Morse EE, Beard J L Haley, NR (1994) Iron deficiency anemia of chronic disease in elderly women: a discriminant analysis approach for differentiation. *Am J Clin Nutr.* 61:590-596.

Allen, RH, Stabler, SP, Savage, D, Lindenbaum, J (1990) Diagnosis of cobalamin deficiency I, Usefulness of serum methylmalonic acid and total homocysteine concentrations. *Am J Hematol* 34:90-98.

American Society of Health System Pharmacists: AHFS Drug Information,(2008) Bethesda, MD, author.

Anderson C, Wochos DN (1982) The utility of serum albumin values in the nutritional assessment of hospitalized patients. *Mayo Clin Proc* 57:181.

Andrews, NC (1999) Disorders of iron metabolism. *N Engl J Med* 341:38-46.

Ascherio, A, Willett, WC, Rimm, EB. (1994) Dietary iron intake and risk of coronary disease among men and women. *Circulation.* 89:969-974.

Ayello E, Thomas D, Litchford M. Nutritional aspects of wound healing. *Home Healthcare Nurse* 1999;17:719-729.

Barclay, L Lie,D. B12, Folate May Reduce Homocysteine Levels Without Affecting Cognition *Am J Clin Nutr.* 2005;82:1320-1326.

Bauer DC, Ettinger B, Browner WS.(1998) Thyroid functions and serum lipids in older women: a population-based study. *Am J Med.* 1998;104:546-551.

Baumgartner, RN, Koehler, KM, Roomero & Garry, P.J (1996) Serum albumin is associated with skeletal muscle in elderly men and women. *AJCN* 64:552-558.

Baxter RC (1986) The somatomedins: Insulin-like growth factors. *Adv Clin Chem* 25:49.

Bernstein LH,(1989) Usefulness of data on albumin and prealbumin concentrations in determining effectiveness of nutritional support. *Clin Chem* 35:271.

Beutler, B (1990) The complex regulation and biology of TNF (cachectin). *Crit Rev* Oncog 2:9.

Blackwell, S & Hendrix,P (2001) Common Anemias: What lies beneath. *Clinician Reviews* 11(3):53-62.

Blake, PG, Flowerdew, G, Blake, RM (1993) Serum albumin in patients on continuous ambulatory peritoneal dialysis. Predictors and correlations with outcomes. ***J Am Soc Nephrol,*** 39:700-706.

Bønaa, KH, Harald, K, (2006) Homocysteine Lowering and Cardiovascular Events after Acute Myocardial Infarction. ***N Engl J Med*** 2006;354.

Bondestam, M, Foucard, T, Mehri, GM (1988) Serum albumin, retinol-binding protein, thyroxin-binding prealbumin and acute phase reactants as indicators of undernutrition in children with undue susceptibility to acute infections. ***Acta Paediatr Scand*** 77:94-98.

Bostom, AG, Shemin, D, Lapane, KL et al (1996) Folate status is the major determinant of fasting total plasma homocysteine levels in maintenance dialysis patients ***Atherosclerosis*** 123:193-202.

Bostom, AG, Shemin, D, Verhoef, P et al (1996) Total plasma homocysteine levels and overall and cardiovascular disease specific mortality in maintenance dialysis patients. ***Circulation*** 94:1-457 (abstract #2671).

Bousney CJ, Beresford, SAA, Omenn, GS, (1995) A quantitative assessment of plasma homocysteine as a risk factor for vascular disease. ***JAMA*** 274:1049-1057.

Brugler, L, Stankovic, A, Berstein, L, Scott, F (2002) The role of visceral protein marketrs in protein calorie malnutrition. ***Clin Chem Lab Med*** 40 (12) 1360-1369.

Campion, EW, deLabry, LO & Glynn (1988) The effect of age on serum albumin in healthy males: report from the Normative Aging Study. ***J Gerontol*** 43(1)M18-20.

Carmel, R (1996) Prevalence of undiagnosed pernicious anemia in the elderly. ***Archives of Internal Medicine*** 156:1097.

Cederholm T, Jagren, C, Hellstrom, K (1995) Outcome of protein-energy malnutrition in elderly medical patients. ***Am J Medical*** 98:67-74.

Chang CG, Adams-Huet B, Provost DA. Acute post-gastric reduction surgery (APGARS) neuropathy. *Obes Surg*. Feb 2004;14(2):182-9.

Cohn, RM & Roth, KS ***Biochemistry and Disease: Bridging Basic Science and clinic I Practice*** (1996) Williams & Wilkins Chapter 18.

Cooper, MJ & Zlotkin, SH (1996) Day to day variation of transferrin receptor and ferritin in healthy men and women. ***AJCN*** 64:738-742.

Corti, MC, Guralnik, JM, Salive, ME, Harris, T, Field, TS, Wallace, RB, (1995) HDL cholesterol predicts heart disease mortality in older persons. ***JAMA*** 274: 539-544.

Coulter, JS (1991) Red blood cell distribution width and mean corpuscular volume: clinical applications. ***Adv Clin Care*** 6(6):13.

Dempsey DT, Multen JL, Buzby GP (1988) The link between nutritional status and clinical outcome: Can nutrition intervention modify it? *Am J Clin Nutr* 47:352.

Deodhar SD (1989) C-reactive protein: The best laboratory indicator available for monitoring disease activity. *Cleve Clin J Med* 56:126.

Diamond I, Messing RO. Neurologic effects of alcoholism. *West J Med*. Sep 1994;161(3):279-87.

Dinarello CA (1992) Biology of interleukin - 1. *Chem Immunol* 51:1.

Dinarello CA, Wolff SM (1993) The role of interleukin - 1 in disease. *N Engl J Med* 328:106.

Erbsloh F, Abel M. Deficiency neuropathies. In: Bruyn GW, Vinken PJ, eds. *Handbook of Clinical Neurology. Vol 7: Diseases of Nerves, Part I.* New York: Wiley Interscience Division; 1970:558-638.

Fischback, F (2008) *A Manual of Laboratory & Diagnostic Tests.* Lippincott: Philadelphia.

Forbes CD, Jackson WF. *A Colour Atlas and Text of Clinical Medicine.* 1993. Aylesbury: Hazell Books Ltd; 428.

Friedman,A, Fadem, S. Reassessment of Albumin as a Nutritional Marker in Kidney Disease. *J Am Soc Nephrol* 21: 223–230, 2010

Fuhrman MP, Charney P, Mueller CM. Hepatic proteins and nutrition assessment. *J Amer Diet Assoc.* 2004;104:1258-1262.

Gallagher-Allred, C., Voss, AC, Finn, S, & McCamish, MA (1996) Malnutrition and clinical outcomes: The case for medical nutrition therapy. *JADA* 96: 366-369.

Gawlikowski J (1992) White cells at war. *AM J Nurs* 92(3):44-51.

Gengenbacher, M Stahelin, HB, Scholer, A, Seiler, WO (2002) Low biochemical nutritional parameters in acutely ill hospitalized elderly patients with and without stage II and IV pressure ulcers. *Aging Cin Exp Res* 14(5): 420-3.

Gill GV, Bell DR. Persisting nutritional neuropathy amongst former war prisoners. *J Neurol Neurosurg Psychiatry.* Oct 1982;45(10):861-5. .

Gomberg-Maitland, M, & William H. Frishman (1998). Thyroid Hormone and Cardiovascular Disease *Am Heart J* 135(2):187-196.

Greenblatt, DJ (1979) Reduced serum albumin concentration in the elderly: a report from the Boston Collaborative Drug Surveillance Program. *JAGS* 27(1) 20-22.

Greenough, WB III, Bennett, RJ (1990) Diarrhea in the elderly, in Hazzard WR, Andres, R, Bierman, EL, Blass, JP (eds): *Principles of Geriatric Medicine and Gerontology,* ed 2. New York: McGraw-Hill 1168-1176.

Guttormsen, A, Schneede, J, Ueland, P, Retsum, H (1996) Kinetics of total plasma homocysteine in subjects with hyperhomocysteinemia due to folate or cobalamin deficiency *Am J Clin Nutr* 63:1914-202.

Hak AE, Pols HA, Visser TJ, Drexhage HA (2000)Subclinical hypothyroidism is an independent risk factor for atherosclerosis and myocardial infarction in elderly women: the Rotterdam Study. *Ann Intern Med*;132:270-278.

Hattori N, Koike H, Sobue G. [Metabolic and nutritional neuropathy]. *Rinsho Shinkeigaku.* Nov 2008;48(11):1026-7.

Hawker, FHA, Stewart, PM, Baxter, RC et al. (1987) Relationship of somatomedin-C/insulin-like growth factor 1 levels to conventional nutritional indices in critically ill patients. *Crit Care Med* 15:732.

Hayek, T, Oiknine, J, Dankner, G, Brook, JG, Aviram, M (1995) HDL apolipo-protein: studies in transgenic mice. *Eur J Cln Chem Clin Biochem.* 33:721-725.

Hine, RJ (1996) What practitioners need to know about folic acid *JADA* 96:451-452.

Ingenbleek, Y, Van Den Schrieck, HG, De Nayer, P, DeVisscher, M (1975) The role of retinol binding protein in protein calorie malnutrition. *Metabolism* 24:633.

Institute of Medicine, Food and Nutrition Board. *Dietary Reference Intakes: Applications in Dietary Planning.* Washington, DC: National Academy Press; 2003.

Institute of Medicine, FNB. *Dietary Reference Intakes for Energy, Carbohydrate, Fiber, Fat, Fatty Acids, Cholesterol, Protein, and Amino Acids.* Food and Nutrition Board. National Academy of Sciences. Washington, DC: National Academy Press; 2002. Available at www.iom.edu/report.asp?id=4340.

Institute of Medicine, FNB. *Dietary Reference Intakes for Vitamin D and Calcium.* Food and Nutrition Board. National Academy of Sciences. Washington, DC: National Academy Press; 2011. Available at www.iom.edu

Iribarren, DM, Reed, CM, Buriel & Dwyer, J.H. (1995). Serum total cholesterol and mortality: Confounding factors and risk modification in Japanese-American men. *JAMA* 273:1926-1932.

Izaka,GJ, Westendorp, RG, Knook, DL (1999) The definition of anemia in older persons. *JAMA* 281:2247-2248.

Jain, SK, McVie, R, Jaramillo, JJ (1996) Effect of modest vitamin E supplementation on blood glycated hemoglobin and triglyceride levels and red cell indices in type I diabetic patients. *AJCN* 64.

Johnson, AM, Merlini,G. Clinical indications for plasma protein assays: transthyretin (prealbumin) in inflammation and malnutrition. *Clin Chem Lab Med* 2007;45(3):419-426

Joosten, E, VandenBerg, A, Riezler, R, Naurath, HJ, Lindembaum, J, Stabler, SP: (1993) Metabolic evidence that deficiencies of vitamin B-12 (Cobalamin), folate and vitamin B-6 occur commonly in elderly people. *Am J Clin Nutr* 58:468-476.

Kee, JL, Hayes, ER (1990) Assessment of patient laboratory data in the acutely ill. **Nurs Clin North Am** 25(4):751-9.

Kesler A, Pianka P. Toxic optic neuropathy. *Curr Neurol Neurosci Rep.* Sep 2003;3(5):410-4.

Kingsbury KJ, Bondy, G (2003) Understanding the essentials of blood lipid metabolism. **Prog Cardiovasc Nurs** 18(1):13-18.

Klonoff-Cohen, H, Barrett-Connor, Edelstein, SL (1992) Albumin levels as a predictor of mortality in the healthy elderly. *J Clin Epidemiol* 45(3) 207-212.

Knoben, JE, Anderson, PO (1988) *Handbook of Clinical Drug Data,* ed 6. Hamilton, IL: Drug Intelligence.

Koehler, KM, Pareo-Tubbeh, SL, Romero, LJ, et al (1997) Folate nutrition and older adults: challenges and opportunities *JADA* 97:167-173.

Koepke, JA, ed.: (1991) *Practical Laboratory Hematology.* New York; Churchill Livingstone.

Koike H, Alcoholic neuropathy. *Curr Opin Neurol.* Oct 2006;19(5):481-6.

Kudsk, KA, Tolley, EA (2003) Albumin as a risk factor in mortality. *JPEN* 27(1)1-9.

Kumar N. Copper deficiency myelopathy (human swayback). *Mayo Clin Proc.* Oct 2006;81(10):1371-84.

Kwiterovich, PO (1997) The effect of dietary fat, antioxidants, and pro-oxidants on blood lipids, lipoproteins and atherosclerosis. *JADA* 97(7):S31-S41.

Lammi-Keef, CJ, Lickteig, ES, Ahluwalia, N, & Haley, R (1996) Day to day variation in iron status indexes is similar for most measures in elderly women with and without rheumatoid arthritis. *JADA* 96(3) 247-251.

Le Quesne PM. Persisting nutritional neuropathy in former war prisoners. *Br Med J (Clin Res Ed).* Mar 19 1983;286(6369):917-8.

Lee GR, Bithell TC, Foerster J, et al., eds.: (1993) *Wintrobe's Clinical Hematology,* ed 9. Philadelphia: Lea & Febiger.

Lewis, CA, Pancharuniti, N, Sauberlich, H: (1992) Plasma folate adequacy as determined by homocysteine level. *Ann NY Acad Sci* 669:360-36.

Li K, McKay G. Images in clinical medicine. Ischemic retinopathy caused by severe megaloblastic anemia. ***N Engl J Med.*** Mar 23 2000;342(12):860.

Linn, BS, Robinson, DS, Limas NG, (1988) Effects of age and nutritional status on surgical outcomes in head and neck cancer. ***Ann Surg.*** 207:267-273.

Lonn,E, Yusuf,S et al. (2006)Homocysteine Lowering with Folic Acid and B Vitamins in Vascular Disease: The Heart Outcomes Prevention Evaluation (HOPE) 2 Investigators ***N Engl J Med*** 2006;351-354.

Looker,AC, Dallman, PR, Carroll, MD et al (1997) Prevalence of iron deficiency in the United States. ***JAMA*** 277:973-976.

Lussier-Cacan, S, Xhignesse, M, Piolog, A, et al (1996) Plasma total homocysteine in healthy subjects: sex specific relation with biological traits. ***AJCN*** 64:587-593.

Makoff, R, Dwyer, J, and Rocco, MV (1996) Folic acid, pyridoxine, cobalamin, and homocysteine and their relationship to cardiovascular disease in end-stage renal disease. ***J Renal Nutrition*** 6:2-11.

Makoff, RK (1995) How much folic acid should be given a dialysis patient? ***Contemporary Dialysis and Nephrology*** November.

Makoff, RK (1996) Micronutrient requirements and replacement in ESRD patients ***Contemporary Dialysis and Nephrology*** August.

Marinella, MA, Market, RJ (1998) Admission serum albumin level and length of hospitalization in elderly patients. ***Am J Med*** 91(9) 851-4.

Massey AC (1992) Microcytic anemia: differential diagnosis and management of iron deficiency anemia. ***Med Clin North Am*** 76:549-566.

Mayer, EL, Jacobsen, DW, Robinson, K (1996) Homocysteine and coronary atherosclerosis. ***J Am Coll Cardiol*** 27:517-527.

Menezes MS, Harada KO, Alvarez G. Painful peripheral polyneuropathy after bariatric surgery. Case reports. ***Rev Bras Anestesiol.*** May-Jun 2008;58(3):252-9.

Meydani, SN, Meydani, M, Blumber, LS et al (1997) Vitamin E supplementation and in vivo immune response in healthy elderly subjects: A randomized controlled trial. ***JAMA*** 277:1380-1386.

Morrison, HI, Schaubel, D, Desmeules, M and Wigle, DT (1996) Serum folate and risk of fatal coronary heart disease ***JAMA*** 275:1893-1896.

Naurath HJ, Joosten, E, Riezler, R, Stabler, SP, Allen RH, L Indenbaum, J: (1995) Effects of vitamin B12, folate, and vitamin B6 supplements in elderly people with normal serum vitamin concentrations. ***Lancet*** 346:85-89.

Newcomer, ME,(2000) Plasma retinol binding protein: structure and function of the prototypic lipoprotein. ***Biochem Biophys Acta*** Oct 18;1482(1-2):57-64.

Nyirenda MJ; Clark DN; Finlayson AR; Read J; Elders A; (2005) Thyroid disease and increased cardiovascular risk. *Thyroid*. 2005; 15(7):718-24.

O'Keefe, CA, Bailey, LB, Thomas, EA, Hofler, SA, (1995) Controlled dietary folate affects folate status in nonpregnant women. *J of Nutrition* 125: 2717-2725.

Pagana, KD, Pagana TJ (2009) *Mosby's Manual of Diagnostic and Laboratory Test Reference.* St. Louis, MO: Mosby.

Pallis CA. Neurological manifestations of nutritional disorders. *Practitioner*. Apr 1974;212(1270 Spec No):509-17.

Pancharuniti, N, Lewis, C,(1994) Plasma homocysteine, folate & vitamin B12 concentrations & risk for early onset coronary artery disease. *AJ CN* 59:940-948.

Paradiso, C (1995) *Fluids and Electrolytes.* Philadelphia, PA: Lippincott.

Patsch, JR, Miesenbock, G,(1992) Relation of triglyceride metabolism and coronary artery disease. *Arterioscler Thromb* 12:1336-1345.

Penninx, BW, Guralnik, JM, Onder, et al (2003) Amenia and decline in physical performance among older persons. *Am J Med* 115(2) 104-110.

Pennypacker, LD, Allen RH, Kelly, JP Matthers, LM (1992) High prevalence of cobalamin deficiency in elderly outpatients. *J Am Geriatr Soc* 40:1197-1204.

Pinchofsky-Devin GD, Kaminski MV (1986) Correlation of pressure sores and nutritional status. *J Am Geriatr Soc* 34:435.

Platania LC, Vogelzang NJ (1990) Interleukin-1: Biology, pathophysiology, and clinical prospects *AM J Med* 89:621.

Poitou Bernert C, Ciangura C. Nutritional deficiency after gastric bypass: diagnosis, prevention and treatment. *Diabetes Metab*. Feb 2007;33(1):13-24.

Prentice, AG, Evans IL (1979) megaloblastic anemia with normal MCV. *Lancet* 1:1606-1607.

Price, SA & Wilson LM (1996) *Pathophysiology clinical Concepts of Disease Processes* Mosby.

Prodan CI, Bottomley SS, Vincent AS, Cowan LD, Copper deficiency after gastric surgery: a reason for caution. *Am J Med Sci*. Apr 2009;337(4):256-8.

Provan D (1999) Mechanism and management of iron deficiency anemia. *Br J Haematol* 105(supplI) :19-26.

Puskarich - May, CL, Sullivan DH, Nelson, CL, Stroope, HF, Walls, RC (1996) The change in serum protein concentration in response to the stress of total joint surgery: A comparison of older versus younger patients. *JAGS* 44:555.

Raisz, LG (2004) Homocysteine and osteoporotic fractures—culprit or bystander? *NEJM* 350:2089-2090.

Rakel RE (1993) **Conn's Current Therapy 1993.** Philadelphia: WB Saunders.
Reed PJ, Laditan AAO (1975) Serum albumin and transferrin in protein-energy malnutrition. **Br J Nutr** 36:255.
Reed, RL, Hepburn, K Adelson, R, Center, B, McKnight, P (2003) Low serum albumin levels, confusion, and fecal incontinence: Are these factors for pressure ulcers in mobility-impaired hospitalized adults. **Gerontology** 49(4)255-256.

Roberts, WL, Paulson, WD (1998) Method specific reference intervals for serum anion gap osmolality. **Clin Chemistry** 44:1528.

Robinson, K, Gupta, A, Dennis, V et al (1996) Hyperhomocysteinemia confers an independent increased risk of atherosclerosis in end-stage renal disease & is closely linked to plasma folate and pyridoxine concentrations. **Circulation** 2743-2448.

Robinson, K, Mayer, EL, Miller, DP, Green, R et al (1995) Hyperhomocysteinemia and low pyridoxal phosphate: common and independent reversible risk factors for coronary artery disease. **Circulation** 92:2825-2830.

Rockey, DC (1999) Occult gastrointestinal bleeding. **N Eng J Med** 341:38-46.

Rosales, FJ, Ross, A. (1998) A Low Molar Ratio of Retinol Binding Protein to Transthyretin Indicates Vitamin A Deficiency during Inflammation: Studies in Rats and A Posteriori Analysis of Vitamin A-Supplemented Children with Measles. **Journal of Nutrition** 128 (10) 1681-1687.

Sachs E, Bernstein LH (1986) Protein markers of nutrition status as related to age and sex. **Clin Chem** 32:339.

Salive, ME, Cornonni-Huntley, J Phillips, CL (1992) Serum albumin in older persons: relationship with age and health status. **J Clin Epidemiol** 45(3)213-221.

Salonen, JT, Nyyssonen, K, Korpela, H, Tuomilehto, J, Seppanen, R, Salonen, R. (1992) High stored iron levels are associated with excess risk of myocardial infarction in Eastern Finnish men, **Circulation** 86:803-811.

Savage, DG, Lindenbaum, JL, Stabler, SP, Allen RH (1994) Sensitivity of serum methylmalonic acid and total homocysteine determinations for diagnosing cobalamin and folate deficiencies. **Am J Med** 96:239-246.

Schnyder, G, Roffi, M, Flammer, Y (2002) Effect of homocysteine-lowering therapy with folic acid, vitamin B12 and vitamin B6 on clinical outcomes after percutaneous coronary intervention: The Swiss Heart Study. **JAMA** 288:973-979.

Shine, JW (1997) Microcytic anemia. **Am Family Physician** 55:2455-2462.

Skikne, BS, Ferguson, B J (990) Serum transferrin receptor distinguishes anemia of chronic disease from iron deficiency. **Blood**. 70: 1955-1958.

Smith FR, Goodman DS, Zaklama JS, et al (1973) Serum vitamin A, retinol-binding protein, and prealbumin concentrations in PCM: I. A functional defect in hepatic retinol release. *Am J Clin Nutr* 26:973.

Smith, FR, Suskind, R, Thanangkul, O Leitzmann, C (1975) Plasma vitamin A, retinol-binding protein and prealbumin concentrations in protein-caloric malnutrition. III. Response to varying dietary treatments *AJCN*, 28,:732-738.

Smith,DL (2000) Anemia in the elderly. *Am Fam Phys* 62:1565-1572.

Spiekerman AM (1987) Laboratory tests for monitoring total parenteral nutrition (TPN) *Clin Chem* 27:1.

Spiekerman AM (1993) Proteins used in nutritional assessment. *Clin Lab Med* 13:1.

Stabler, SP (1995) Screening the older population for cobalamin (Vitamin B12) deficiency *J Am Geriatr Soc* 43:1290-1297.

Starker PM, Gump FE, Askanazi J, et al (1982) Serum albumin levels as an index of nutritional support. *Surgery* 91:194.

Stein, JH, McBride, PE (1998) Hyperhomocysteinemia & atherosclerosis vascular disease: pathophysiology, screening & treatment. *Arch Intern Med*, 158:1301-1306.

Steinberg, D (1995) Clinical trials of antioxidants in atherosclerosis: are we doing the right thing? *Lancet* 346:36-38.

Stewart, SH, Mainous, A (2002) Relation between alcohol consumption and C-reactive protein in the adult population. *J Am Board Fam Pract* 15(6): 437-442.

Tanyel MC, Mancano LD. Neurologic findings in vitamin E deficiency. *Am Fam Physician*. Jan 1997;55(1):197-201.

Thaisetthawatkul P, Collazo-Clavell ML, Sarr MG, Norell JE, Dyck PJ. A controlled study of peripheral neuropathy after bariatric surgery. *Neurology*. Oct 26 2004;63(8):1462-70.

Thomas, S; Wolf, S; Murphy, K,; Chinkes, D (2004) The Long-Term Effect of Oxandroloneon Hepatic Acute Phase Proteins in Severely Burned Children. *Journal of Trauma-Injury Infection & Critical Care*. 56(1):37-44.

Tucker, KL, Selhub, J, Wilson, PWF & Rosenbeug, IH (1996) Dietary intake pattern relates to plasma folate and homocysteine concentrations in the Framingham Heart Study. *Journal of Nutrition*. 126:3025-3031.

U.S. Preventive Services Task Force. *Screening Thyroid Disease: Recommendation Statement*. January 2004. Agency for Healthcare Research and Quality, Rockville, MD.
http://www.ahrq.gov/clinic/3rduspstf/thyroid/thyrrs.htm

Ubbink, A, VanderMeerwe, R (1996) The effect of subnormal vitamin B6 status on homocysteine metabolism. ***Journal of Clinical Investigation.*** 98:177-184.

VanAsselt, DZ, VanderBroek (1996) Free and protein cobalamin absorption in healthy middle-aged and older subjects. ***JAGS*** 44:949-953.

Vassall, P (1992) The pathophysiology of tumor necrosis factors. ***Annu Rev Immunol*** 10:411.

Verdery RB, Golbderg, AP (1991) Hypocholesterolemia as a predictor of death: A prospective study of 224 nursing home residents. ***J Gerontol Med Sci*** 46:M84.

Warren, JL, Bacon WE, Harris, T (1991) The burden and outcomes associated with dehydration among US elderly. ***Am J Public Health***, 84:1265-1269.

Weber GA, Sloan P, Davies D. Nutritionally-induced peripheral neuropathies. *Clin Podiatr Med Surg*. Jan 1990;7(1):107-28.

Winkler MF, Gerrior SA, Pomp A, Albina JE (1980) Use of retinol-binding protein and prealbumin as indicators of the response to nutritional therapy. ***J Am Diet Assoc.*** 89:684.

Yao, Y, Yao, SL (1992) Prevalence of vitamin B_{12} deficiency among geriatric outpatients. ***Journal Family Practice*** 35:524-528.

Young, DS (1987) Implementation of SI Units for clinical laboratory data. ***Annals of Internal Medicine.*** 10: 114-129.

Zeman, F & Ney D (1996) ***Applications in Medical Nutritional Therapy.*** Englewood Cliff, NJ: Prentice Hall.

Zittoun, JA, Cooper, BA (1989) ***Folates and Cobalamins.*** Spring-Verlag: Berlin, Germany.

INDEX

5'-nucleotidase, 58-9, 80, 88
5-fluorouracil, 127, 146
Abacavir, 54, 81, 157
Abarelix, 277
Acarbose, 54, 81, 88, 119, 159, 170, 176, 278
ACE inhibitors, 95, 133, 215, 257, 278
Acebutolol, 54, 60, 81, 119, 133, 157, 193
Acetaminophen, 54, 60, 80, 81, 88, 95, 133, 156-7, 159, 160, 236, 255
Acetanilid, 172
Acetazolamide, 64, 88, 95, 105, 109, 112, 157, 159, 169, 198, 210, 216, 219, 236, 255, 257
Acetohexamide, 54, 60, 81, 88, 92, 118, 133, 159
Acetophenazine, 88, 92, 118
Acetylcysteine, 112
Acetylsalicylic acid, 128, 150, 189, 277-8
Achlorhydria, 41, 286
Acidosis, 73-7, 109, 112, 171-2, 197, 205, 207, 209, 214, 219, 260
Acromegaly, 95, 104, 132, 133, 137, 156, 163, 165, 166, 169, 176, 209, 269
ACTH, 118, 123, 156, 189, 190
Acute renal failure, 78, 80, 256
Acute tubular necrosis, 95, 130, 131, 133, 193
Acyclovir, 54, 60, 62, 81, 88, 95, 133
Addison's disease, 123, 163, 166, 197, 210, 219, 252-3, 257, 295
Adefovir 54, 81, 133
Adenocarcinoma, 126
Adenosine, 157
Adrenal insufficiency, 178
Adrenalin, 295
Adrenocortical hypofunction/insufficiency, 205, 246, 257
Afibrinogenemia, 146
AIDS, 44, 118, 178, 182, 189, 223, 227, 232, 277, 282, 294, 296
Alanine aminotransferase (ALT), 21, 53-7, 59, 64, 80, 126, 192
Albendazole, 54, 60, 81, 88, 95, 133
Albumin, 17, 21, 33, 35, 220-237
Albuterol, 119, 127, 157, 198, 210, 216
Alcohol/ Alcoholism, 64, 71, 104, 118, 121, 127, 155, 157, 175, 193, 197, 215, 246, 260, 277, 284, 286
Aldesleukin, 54, 60, 81, 88, 95, 104-5, 119, 133, 157, 159, 198, 210, 215-6, 236, 254
Aldosterone/ Aldosteronism, 77-8, 112-3, 207, 213, 215, 219, 256
Alendronate, 62, 105, 110, 210
Alkaline antacids, 95, 104, 133, 198, 210
Alkaline phosphatase (ALP), 53, 58-62, 64, 80, 88, 126, 192, 288
Alkalosis, 73-75, 103, 111, 209
Allopurinol, 54, 60, 81, 85, 88, 92, 95, 113, 119, 150, 159, 189, 239, 295
Alprazolam, 54, 60, 81, 88, 133, 135
Altretamine, 95, 133
Aluminium, 104, 210
Aluminum antacids, 62

Amantadine, 95
Amifostine, 105
Amikacin 91, 95, 97, 119, 128, 133, 135, 194, 236
Amiloride, 88, 95, 109, 113, 119, 133, 198, 215, 219, 254, 255, 257
Aminocaproic acid, 127, 215
Aminoglutethimide, 54, 60, 81, 88, 118, 124, 215, 255
Aminoglycosides, 131, 236, 286
Aminophylline, 157, 236
Aminosalicylic acid, 54, 60, 81, 88, 92, 119, 150, 157, 169, 216, 236, 239, 286
Amiodarone, 54, 60, 70, 81, 88, 95, 118-9, 133, 157, 193, 223, 228, 265, 266, 271-3, 275, 277-8
Amitriptyline, 54, 60, 81, 88, 157
Amlodipine, 105, 119, 210, 216, 278
Ammonia, 21, 63-65, 93, 94, 198
Ammonium chloride 64, 109, 112, 133, 198, 215, 216, 219, 255, 257
Amoxapine, 54, 60, 81, 88, 112, 127, 133, 157
Amphetamine, 123, 159, 275
Amphotericin, 54, 60, 81, 88, 95, 105, 112, 118, 127, 133, 157, 193, 198, 215, 216, 236, 255
Ampicillin, 54, 60, 81, 119, 127, 150, 157, 169, 170, 236, 254
Amprenavir, 118
Amrinone, 54, 60, 81, 88
Amyl nitrite, 95
Amyloidosis, 59, 131, 207, 234, 235
Anabolic steroids, 54, 60, 81, 88, 95, 104, 118, 131, 137, 146, 159, 193, 210, 223, 228, 239, 254, 266, 269, 272-3, 275, 278, 299
Anastrazole, 54, 60, 81, 88, 118
Androgens, 70, 124, 223, 228
Anemia of chronic and inflammatory diseases, 41-44, 139
Anesthesia, 156
Angina, 79, 99, 180, 262
Angioplasty, 80
Anistreplase, 146
Anorexia nervosa, 70, 149, 277
Antacids, 41, 62, 95, 104, 109, 133, 148, 150, 196-8, 210
Anterior pituitary hypofunction, 246
Antibiotics, 60, 92, 118, 179, 182, 198, 219, 294, 295
Anticonvulsants, 47, 54, 60, 81, 88, 91, 105, 109, 123, 140, 148, 150, 194, 210, 249, 286, 295
Antidepressants, 157
Antifungal agents, 54, 60, 81, 88, 150
Antihistamines, 295
Antihypertensives, 118
Antimalarials, 47, 88, 148, 172
Antimetabolites, 295
Antineoplastic, 179, 182, 292, 296
Antipyretics, 88, 172
Antithyroid, 62, 144, 295
Aplastic anemia, 188, 246, 295
Apolipoprotein A, (Apo A) 66-71

Apo A-1/ Apo B ratio, 66-71
Apolipoprotein B, (Apo B), 66-71
Apo C-II deficiency, 70, 121
Apolipoprotein E, (Apo E), 66-71
Aprepitant 54, 81, 95
Ardeparin, 54, 60, 81, 277
Aripiprazole 54, 81, 95, 127, 157, 194, 215, 265
Arrhythmias, 127
Arsenic, 54, 60, 62, 81, 95, 105, 198, 216, 236, 295
Arterial blood gases (ABGs), 72-8
Ascites, 34, 130, 204, 205, 215, 277, 232, 252-3
Ascorbic acid, (Vitamin C) 85, 88, 92, 97, 109, 113, 119, 128, 131, 133, 135, 137, 144, 159-60, 169, 170, 172, 194, 236, 249, 277, 278, 286
Asparaginase, 54, 60, 64, 81, 88, 95, 105, 112, 118, 119, 133, 146, 157, 169, 236, 269, 275, 278
Aspartate aminotransferase (AST), 21, 53, 59, 64, 79-85, 88, 126, 192
Aspirin, 57, 88, 91, 95, 105, 112, 118, 119, 121, 123, 127, 134, 140, 150, 157, 159, 169, 170, 172, 176, 179, 182, 189, 194, 198, 210, 216, 219, 236, 257, 266, 271, 273, 275, 295
Atazanavir, 88, 118, 157
Atenolol, 70, 95, 118, 119, 134, 135, 146, 157, 159, 176, 203, 215, 237, 257, 265, 275, 277
Atherosclerosis, 67-8, 118, 129, 133, 183-4
Atomoxetine 54, 81, 89
Atorvastatin, 54, 60, 70, 81, 89, 119, 127, 278
Atovaquone, 54, 60, 81, 255
Atrophic gastritis, 49, 286
Atropine, 123, 157, 159
Auranofin, 54, 60, 81, 89, 194, 236
Aurothioglucose, 54, 60, 81, 236
Autoimmune disease, 138, 287, 292, 294, 297
Azaribine, 185
Azathioprine, 54, 60, 62, 81, 89, 95, 118-9, 134, 157, 198, 210, 215-6, 278
Azithromycin, 54, 60, 81, 89, 95, 127, 134, 157, 194, 210, 215-6
Azlocillin, 169
Azotemia, 63, 80, 93, 133, 205, 257
Aztreonam, 54, 60, 81, 95, 134
B12 deficiency, 44-50, 148-9, 183, 185, 199-200, 240, 247-9, 285
B6 deficiency, 80, 149, 185, 188
Bacitracin, 95, 236
Baclofen, 157
Bacterial meningitis, 100
Barbiturates, 54, 60, 64, 77, 81, 89, 91, 92, 124, 134, 150, 239, 295
Bariatric procedures, 260, 286, 288-90, 299
Barium chloride poisoning 215
Barium, 54, 60, 81, 215
Bartter's syndrome, 215, 219, 257
Basiliximab, 104, 105, 118, 157, 159, 198, 210, 215, 216, 236
Basophils, 291-296
BCG vaccine, 54, 60, 81, 89
Beclomethasone, 118, 124, 157

Benazepril, 54, 60, 82, 89, 95, 134, 157, 159, 203, 215, 236, 255
Benzthiazide, 89, 95, 134, 169, 216, 257
Bepridil, 54, 60, 82
Beriberi, 80, 259-60
Beta blockers, 70, 118, 176, 277
Betamethasone, 124, 157, 216, 219, 254
Betaxolol, 54, 60, 82, 95, 118, 134, 157, 194, 215, 216, 236
Bevacizumab, 89, 216
Bicalutamide, 54, 82, 89, 118, 134, 146, 157
Bicarbonate, 72-78, 104, 110-1, 113, 214, 236
Biliary cirrhosis, 59, 118, 121
Biliary obstruction, 59, 70, 80
Bilirubin, 21-2, 86-92, 225
Bisacodyl, 170, 216
Bismuth subsalicylate, 89, 95, 169, 236
Bisoprolol, 54, 70, 82, 95, 118, 120, 134, 157, 210, 215, 277-8
Bisphosphonates, 105, 110
Bitolterol, 54, 60, 82
Bladder outlet obstruction, 95
Bladder tumors, 235
Bleomycin, 89
Blind loop syndrome, 149, 249
Blood urea nitrogen (BUN), 33, 35, 74, 76, 93-7, 130, 133, 137
Bone cancer 59, 109
Bone disease, 59
Bone marrow failure, 178, 246
Bone metastasis, 103, 209
Bortezomib, 110, 216
Breast cancer, 103, 139, 144, 207
Bromocriptine, 54, 60, 82
Budesonide, 124, 157
Bumetanide, 109, 113, 198, 216, 219, 257
Bupropion, 54, 60, 82, 89, 169
Burkitt's lymphoma, 104
Burns, 54, 81, 95, 112, 118, 121, 131, 151, 178, 182, 189, 214, 215, 223, 227, 231-2, 253, 298
Busulfan, 54, 60, 82, 89, 95
Caffeine, 91, 153, 155, 159, 166
Calcitonin, 62, 105, 109, 110, 157, 198, 210, 219, 257, 265
Calcitriol, 54, 60, 62, 82, 96, 104, 118, 198, 210, 236
Calcium, 22, 58, 101-10, 159, 195, 198, 208, 213, 226, 287
Cancer, 101-3, 109, 118, 122, 132, 142, 144, 146, 182, 188, 192, 227, 271, 275
Candesartan, 54, 60, 82, 89, 96, 127, 134, 157, 215-6
Cannabis, 96, 112, 135, 157, 215, 254
Capecitabine, 54, 60, 82
Capreomycin, 60, 96, 97, 134, 216, 236
Captopril, 60, 70, 89, 96, 104, 118, 120, 127, 131, 134-5, 137, 157, 159, 169, 194, 203, 215-6, 237, 255, 257, 278
Carbamazepine, 54, 60, 69, 82, 89, 91, 96, 105, 112, 118, 134, 140, 169, 185, 210, 216, 219, 236, 254-5, 257, 265-6, 269, 271-3, 277, 288

Carbenicillin, 54, 60, 82, 89, 127, 169, 194, 216, 219, 254
Carbon dioxide, 72-78, 180
Carbon monoxide (CO) poisoning, 77, 127, 131
Cardiac aneurysm, 126
Cardiac catheterization, 80
Cardiac defibrillation, 127
Cardiac ischemia, 126
Cardiac surgery, 80
Carmustine, 54, 60, 82, 89, 112
Carteolol, 127, 203
Cartilage-hair hypoplasia, 295
Carvedilol, 57, 60, 62, 89, 96, 112, 118, 120, 134, 157, 159, 169, 216, 236, 255, 257, 277-8
Cascara, 216
Casodex, 277
Caspofungin, 134
Castor oil, 236
Cathartics, 216, 255
Cefaclor, 96, 134, 169, 236
Cefadroxil, 134
Cefamandole, 96, 134, 146, 169, 236
Cefazolin, 89, 96, 134, 169
Cefdinir, 89, 157, 159, 169, 194, 210, 215, 236
Cefepime, 134, 169
Cefixime, 65, 96, 134, 169
Cefonicid, 96, 194
Cefoperazone, 89, 96, 134, 169
Cefotaxime, 65, 96, 97, 104, 112, 113, 118, 127, 134, 157, 189, 194, 198, 210, 215, 254
Cefotetan, 96, 134, 194
Cefoxitin, 89, 96, 131, 134, 137, 194
Cefpodoxime, 89, 96, 134, 157, 159, 194
Cefprozil, 134
Ceftazidime, 89, 96, 134, 194
Ceftibuten, 89, 96, 134
Ceftizoxime, 89,96, 127, 134
Ceftriaxone, 89, 96, 134
Cefuroxime, 89, 96, 134, 157, 159, 169, 194
Celiac disease, 59, 94, 104, 148, 149, 166, 241, 288
Centers for Medicare (CMS), 14
Cephalexin, 96, 134, 169, 216
Cephaloridine, 134, 236
Cephalosporin, 54, 60, 82, 131, 137, 169
Cephalothin, 89, 96, 131, 134, 137, 140, 236, 239
Cephapirin, 140
Cephradine, 134
Cerebral infarction, 80
Cerebrovascular accident (CVA) 125, 126, 156, 169, 193
Cerebrovascular disease, 126, 183, 185
Cerivastatin, 54, 60, 82, 89, 127, 278
Cetirizine, 54, 60, 82, 89, 96, 134

Chediak-Higashi syndrome, 295
Chemotherapy, 62, 96, 146, 214, 292-296
Chenodiol, 54, 60, 82, 89, 118, 278
Chloral hydrate, 54, 82, 89, 170, 236, 239, 249, 286
Chlorambucil, 54, 82, 89, 120, 135
Chloramphenicol, 54, 60, 82, 89, 97, 150, 157, 159, 179, 182, 189, 190, 194, 239, 294
Chlordane, 89, 127, 194, 277
Chlordiazepoxide, 54, 60, 82, 89, 127
Chlorhexidine, 92, 236
Chloride, 22, 28, 73, 111-13, 181
Chloroform, 60, 89, 96, 120, 127, 236, 295
Chloroquine, 89, 105, 110, 159, 216
Chlorothiazide, 54, 77, 82, 89, 96, 104, 105,109, 110, 112, 118, 127, 134, 157, 169, 198, 216, 255, 257, 277
Chlorpheniramine, 54, 60, 82, 96, 112, 169, 236
Chlorpromazine, 54, 60, 82, 89, 92, 118, 127, 157, 159, 169, 194, 236, 249, 265, 286
Chlorpropamide, 54, 60, 82, 89, 104, 113, 118, 120, 134, 159, 194, 236, 255
Chlortetracycline, 54, 82, 89, 96, 194
Chlorthalidone, 54, 64, 70, 82, 96, 104, 113, 118, 120, 127, 134, 157, 169, 194, 198, 203, 216, 219, 236, 254, 255, 257, 277, 278
Chlorzoxazone, 54, 60, 82, 89
Cholestasis, 53, 69, 88, 92, 118, 121
Cholesterol, 14, 22, 67, 68, 114-121, 121, 185, 262, 277
Cholestyramine, 54, 70, 82, 109, 113, 120, 127, 150, 157, 159, 170, 189, 239, 249, 254, 275, 277-8, 286
Choline magnesium trisalicylate, 54, 82
Chronic blood loss, 28, 39, 41, 172, 175, 189, 190, 240, 243
Chronic pulmonary disease, (COPD), 74, 77-8, 118, 121, 130, 178, 182, 277
Chronic renal failure, 44, 69, 71, 127, 138-9, 141, 149, 156, 163, 165-6, 175, 196, 200, 206, 279, 288, 298
Cidofovir, 54, 60, 82, 89, 105, 134, 157, 169, 216, 236
Cilazapril, 120
Cilostazol, 237
Cimetidine, 54, 60, 82, 89, 96, 131, 134, 137, 159, 194, 239, 275
Cinacalcet, 105
Cinoxacin, 54, 60, 82, 96, 134
Ciprofloxacin, 54, 60, 82, 96, 134, 159, 194
Cirrhosis, alcoholic, 80, 192, 277, 281
Cirrhosis, hepatic 53, 59, 80-1, 88, 103, 121, 130, 143, 146, 149, 156, 165, 178, 182, 190, 192, 207, 231, 238, 239, 246, 271, 275, 282, 299
Cisplatin, 54, 82, 89, 96, 105, 110, 131, 134, 137, 189, 198, 210, 215-6, 236, 255, 257
CK-BB, 125-8
CK-MB, 125-8, 279
CK-MM, 125-8
Cladribine, 54, 82, 89
Clarithromycin, 54, 82, 96, 134

Clindamycin, 54, 60, 82, 89, 96, 127, 134, 194, 236
Clofarabine, 54, 82, 89, 134
Clofazimine, 54, 82, 89
Clofibrate, 54, 60, 62, 82, 89, 118, 120, 127, 134, 146, 157, 159, 194, 215, 236, 239, 255, 257, 266, 269, 272, 273, 275, 278
Clomiphene, 54, 82, 120, 265, 275
Clomipramine, 54, 82, 85, 123, 275
Clonidine, 54, 60, 82, 89, 96, 118, 120, 124, 127, 134, 157, 203, 254-5
Clopidogrel, 55, 82, 89, 118
Clorazepate, 55, 82, 96, 109, 134
Clotrimazole, 96
Cloxacillin, 55, 82
Clozapine, 55, 60, 82, 89, 127, 140, 157, 255
Cobalt, 248
Cocaine, 126
Codeine, 55, 82, 96, 134, 159, 194, 236
Coenzyme Q10, 120
Colchicine, 54, 60, 62, 82, 89, 120, 127, 150, 157, 189, 249, 277, 286
Colestipol, 55, 60, 70, 82, 120, 269, 278
Colistimethate, 134
Colistin, 96, 134, 236
Collagen vascular diseases, 143, 188
Colloid osmotic pressure, 34
Colon cancer, 107, 139
Congenital heart disease, 178, 182
Congestive heart failure (CHF), 34, 44, 80, 94, 130, 138, 181-2, 193, 201-2, 207, 252, 254, 256, 262
Conjugated estrogens,60, 89, 118, 120, 265, 272-3
Convulsions, 80, 126, 156
Coronary artery disease (CAD), 99, 114-7, 141, 145-6, 262
Coronary heart disease, 114-8
Corticosteroids, 105, 109, 113, 119, 124, 131, 137, 157, 169, 216, 219, 223, 228, 236, 254, 257, 266, 269, 272-3, 275
Corticotropin, 109, 113, 123, 140, 157, 169, 189, 216, 219, 236, 269
Cortisol, 122-4, 228
Cortisone, 55, 82, 105, 113, 119, 123, 140, 157, 189, 216, 219, 254, 257, 269
Cotrimoxazole, 96, 134, 275
Coumadin, 89
Cranial pressure, 104, 169
C-Reactive protein (CRP), 17, 98-100, 117, 138, 220, 221-3, 225-6
Creatine kinase (CK), 53, 59, 79, 80, 125-8, 192, 279
Creatine phosphokinase CPK, 125-8
Creatinine clearance, 24, 129-31, 133
Creatinine, 15, 22, 36-7, 49, 74, 93-4, 107, 129-37, 184, 199, 233
Cretinism, 264, 271, 272, 274
Crigler-Najjar syndrome, 88
Crohn's disease, 44, 49, 100, 149, 227, 249, 299
Crushing injuries, 127, 214
Cushing's disease or syndrome , 70, 122-3, 156, 163-4, 176, 227, 251, 253, 256, 271, 275, 295
Cyclobenzaprine, 55, 60, 82, 89, 157, 169

Cyclophosphamide, 55, 60, 82, 89, 119, 140, 157, 169, 255
Cycloserine, 60, 89, 150, 284
Cyclosporine, 57, 60, 85, 89, 91, 96, 113, 119, 134, 140, 157, 198, 203, 215, 236, 257, 277
Cyclothiazide, 257
Cyproheptadine, 55, 60, 82, 89
Cystic fibrosis, 76, 156, 215, 221, 281, 282, 288, 290
Cytarabine, 55, 60, 82, 89, 255
Cytomegalovirus, 59
Dacarbazine, 55, 82, 89
Dactinomycin, 60, 82, 89
Dalfopristin, 194, 216
Dalteparin, 55, 82
Danazol, 55, 60, 62, 82, 119, 124, 127, 134, 146, 157, 215, 266, 269, 271, 273, 275, 277-8
Dantrolene, 55, 82, 89, 119, 127-8, 236
Dapsone, 55, 60, 82, 89, 92, 119, 127, 172, 194, 255
Deferoxamine, 144, 176, 189
Dehydration, 29-33, 93-4, 109, 112, 129, 131, 133, 155-6, 178, 181, 189, 197, 204-5, 207, 215, 223, 226, 232, 239, 251-3, 256, 258
Delirium tremens, 126, 193
Demeclocycline, 55, 60, 82, 96, 134
Dermatomyositis 80, 126
Dermatomyositis, 80, 126
Desipramine, 55, 60, 82, 89, 157, 159, 236
Desmopressin, 55, 82, 255
Dexamethasone, 96, 109, 124, 127-8, 140, 157, 169, 215-6, 219, 257, 275
Dexfenfluramine, 278
Dexrazoxane, 134
Dextran, 96, 119, 134, 140, 146, 157, 189, 228
Dextroamphetamine, 124, 157, 159, 169
Dextrose IV infusions, 157, 168
Dextrothyroxine, 89, 157, 170
Diabetes insipidus, 31, 112, 205-7, 251, 253, 258
Diabetes mellitus, 29, 59, 69-70, 95, 100, 137, 151-70, 173-76, 197, 215, 233-5, 248, 258, 276-7, 298
Diabetes, gestational(GDM) 154-6, 161-2, 165, 168, 175
Diabetic acidosis 197, 219, 254
Diabetic glomerulosclerosis, 234
Diabetic ketoacidosis (DKA), 95, 209
Diabetic nephropathy, 133, 234
Diaphoresis, 30, 197, 256
Diarrhea, 31, 33, 48, 76-8, 112, 148, 178, 182, 197, 210, 214, 253, 258, 260, 281-2, 290
Diazepam, 55, 60, 82, 89, 96, 109, 119, 159, 170
Diazoxide, 55, 60, 82, 89, 96, 113, 123-4, 157, 159, 169-70, 219, 236, 254, 257
Diclofenac, 55, 60, 82, 89, 96, 119, 123, 127, 134, 157, 194, 255, 275
Dicloxacillin, 89
Dicumarol, 55, 82, 238
Didanosine, 55, 60, 82, 89, 127, 134, 157, 277

Dienestrol, 55, 82, 89, 104
Diethylstilbestrol, 55, 82, 89, 104, 150, 157, 269
Differential Count, 291-7
Diflunisal, 55, 82, 89
Digitalis, 239, 257
Digoxin, 127, 170, 198, 215, 216
Dihydrotachysterol, 105, 236
Diltiazem, 55, 60, 82, 89, 109, 120, 127, 157, 159, 176, 194, 278
Dimercaprol, 89, 109, 157, 159
Diphenhydramine, 65, 89, 239
Diphenoxylate, 157
Dipyridamole, 203, 210, 237
Disopyramide, 55, 60, 82, 89, 96, 134, 159
Disseminated intravascular coagulation (DIC), 145-6, 239
Disulfiram, 55, 60, 82, 89, 119
Diuretics, 31, 33, 63, 70, 77, 92, 96, 105, 127, 134, 172, 215-6, 219, 255, 295
Diverticulosis, 188
Dobutamine, 120, 135, 157, 216
Docetaxel, 55, 60, 82, 89
Donepezil, 127, 157, 194, 216
Dopamine, 134-5, 157, 266
Doxapram, 236
Doxazosin, 70, 120, 159, 216, 278
Doxepin, 89, 157, 159, 255, 257
Doxorubicin, 55, 60, 82, 89, 96, 105, 134, 157, 159, 169, 194, 198, 203, 210, 215-6, 236, 254, 255
Doxycycline, 55, 60, 82, 89, 96, 134, 236, 255
Dronabinol, 55, 82
Droperidol, 128
Dubin-Johnson syndrome, 88, 92
Duloxetine, 89, 159
Dysfibrinogenemia, 146
Eclampsia, 112, 146, 178, 182, 296
Eczema, 297
Edema, 34-5, 77, 207, 227, 233, 252, 254, 258, 260, 262
Efavirenz, 119
Electroconvulsive therapy, 126
Electromyography, 127
Eletriptan, 55, 82, 85
Emphysema, pulmonary, 64, 77-8, 113, 229, 256
Enalapril, 55, 60, 82, 89, 96, 119-20, 134, 157, 159, 169, 176, 194, 215-6, 236-7, 257, 277-8
Encephalopathy, 63-4, 87, 156, 260
End stage renal disease, 46, 137, 144, 183
Endocarditis, 44, 231
Endocrine disorders, 156, 169
Enflurane, 134
Enfuvirtide, 157, 277
Enoxacin, 55, 82
Enoxaparin, 55, 82, 89, 271, 273

Eosinophilia-myalgia syndrome, 126
Eosinophils, 291-7
Ephedra, 157
Ephedrine, 124, 157, 169
Epinephrine, 89, 119, 151, 157, 166, 283, 295
Epirubicin, 236
Eplerenone, 55, 82, 96, 119, 134, 215, 236, 255
Epoetin alfa, 96, 134, 210, 215
Epoprostenol, 216
Eprosartan, 96, 134
Ergocalciferol, 109, 287
Ergot preparations, 96, 236
Erlotinib, 55, 82, 89
Erythematous, 182
Erythroblastosis fetalis, 88, 245
Erythrocyte sedimentation rate, (ESR) 51, 100, 138-40, 221, 223, 226
Erythrocytosis, 178
Erythromycin, 55, 60, 82, 89, 120, 150, 159
Erythropoietin, 105, 203, 210, 215, 269, 271, 273, 275
Escitalopram, 89, 119, 157
Esomeprazole, 255
Esomeprazole, 255
Estramustine, 89, 105, 194, 210
Estrogen, 55, 60, 62, 68-71, 82, 89, 105, 110, 118, 120, 121, 123, 146, 157, 170, 189, 223, 228, 239, 254, 265, 269, 272, 273, 277, 278
Estropipate, 55, 61, 82, 89, 105, 146, 150, 157, 275
Ethacrynic acid, 109, 157, 159, 169, 198, 216, 219, 255, 257
Ethambutol, 55, 61, 82, 89, 96, 134
Ethanol, 69-70, 119, 189, 204-5
Ethchlorvynol, 55, 82, 127
Ether, 55, 61, 82, 89, 96, 119, 123, 169, 236
Ethionamide, 61, 89, 157, 169
Ethosuximide, 89, 96, 236
Etidocaine, 127
Etidronate, 62, 96, 105, 110, 134, 210
Etodolac, 55, 82, 92, 257
Etoposide, 55, 82, 89
Etretinate, 55, 61, 70, 82, 89, 96, 105, 113, 119, 127, 134, 140, 157, 159, 169, 194, 210, 215, 216, 236, 254, 255, 277
Euthyroidism sick disease, 265
Excess fluid intake, 207
Excess vitamin B ingestion, 59
Exercise, 67, 76, 100, 116, 120, 125, 130, 156, 166, 174, 233
Extracellular fluid, 33-4, 212, 250-1
Factitious hyperthyroidism, 265, 271-2, 275
Factor IX, 89, 238-9
Factor VIIa, 146
Familial HDL lipoproteinemia, 121
Familial hyperalphalipoproteinemia, 69
Familial hypertriglyceridemia, 69
Familial hypoalphalipoproteinemia, 69

Familial hypolipoproteinemia, 121
Familial idiopathic dysproteinemia, 227
Famotidine, 55, 61, 82, 89, 105
Fanconi syndrome, 169
Fat embolism, 103
Fava beans, 171
Felbamate, 55, 64, 82, 89, 105, 157, 159, 216
Felodipine, 61, 157, 198, 215, 219, 257
Fenfluramine, 159
Fenofibrate, 55, 70, 82, 89, 120, 127, 146, 157, 159, 278
Fenoldopam, 109, 219, 257, 266
Fenoprofen, 55, 61, 82, 89, 96, 123, 134, 194, 236
Ferritin, 17, 22, 39, 42, 45-7, 50-1, 141-4, 178, 181, 186-8, 299
Ferrous sulfate, 144, 170, 265
Fever, 29-32, 44, 95, 98, 100, 127, 139, 258, 295
Fibrinogen, 17, 27, 100, 138, 145-6, 238
Fibrinolysins, 146
Fish eye disease, 69
Flaxseed oil, 278
Flecainide, 55, 61, 82
Floxuridine, 194
Fluconazole, 55, 61, 82, 89, 216, 277
Flucytosine, 55, 61, 82, 89, 96, 134, 159, 216
Fludarabine, 96, 134
Fludrocortisone 157, 169, 216, 219, 254
Fluorides, 190, 194
Fluorouracil, 55, 61, 82, 89, 127, 146, 275
Fluoxetine, 255
Fluoxymesterone, 55, 61, 82, 89, 105, 119, 120, 134, 157, 159, 269
Fluphenazine, 55, 61, 82, 89, 92, 194
Flurazepam, 55, 61, 82, 89, 159, 170
Flutamide, 55, 61, 82, 89, 96
Fluvastatin, 55, 61, 82, 89, 120, 127, 140, 146, 277-8
Fluvoxamine, 55, 82, 119, 157, 159, 194, 216, 255
Folate or Folic Acid, 22, 44-50, 147-50, 183-5, 200, 240, 247, 283, 286
Fosamprenavir 157, 277
Foscarnet, 55, 61, 82, 96, 105, 127, 134, 157, 159, 169, 194, 198, 210, 216, 236, 255
Fosinopril, 55, 82, 89, 119, 120, 157, 159, 216, 237
Fosphenytoin, 55, 61, 82, 89, 157, 215, 216, 254
Free Thyroxine Index (FTI), 261-275
Fructose intolerance, 156
Furazolidone, 55, 83, 89, 170
Furosemide, 55, 64, 69, 70, 82, 90, 96, 105, 109, 113, 119, 123, 127, 134, 157, 159, 170, 194, 198, 210, 216, 236-7, 255, 257, 271, 273, 275, 277
Gabapentin, 96, 119, 134, 170, 236
Galactosemia, 156, 235
Gallium, 105
Gallstones, 87, 88, 92
Ganciclovir, 55, 61, 83, 90, 96, 127, 134, 157, 159, 194, 216
Gangrene, 80, 138

Garlic, 55, 83
Gastrectomy, 165, 167, 241, 286
Gemcitabine, 55, 61, 83, 90, 96, 134, 236
Gemfibrozil, 55, 61, 69-70, 83, 90, 120, 123, 127, 134, 146, 157, 159, 176, 278
Gentamicin, 55, 61, 83, 90, 96, 105, 131, 134, 137, 179, 182, 194, 198, 216, 219, 236, 255
Gigantism, 132, 133, 156
Gilbert's syndrome, 59, 88
Glimepiride, 55, 61, 83, 90, 157, 159, 176, 216, 255
Glipizide, 159, 176
Globulin, 186, 220-232, 261-275
Glomerulonephritis, 95, 118, 121, 130-1, 133, 146, 193, 219, 233-5, 258
Glucagon, 151-152, 155-157, 168, 175
Glucagonoma, 156, 166, 170, 176
Glucocorticoids, 105, 275, 277
Glucosamine, 157, 159
Glucose Tolerance Test, Oral (GTT), 155, 162, 165-167, 175
Glucose, 22, 29, 54, 60, 81, 122-3, 151-170, 173-175, 205, 208-9, 214, 217, 253, 258-9, 283
Glucose-6-Phosphate Dehydrogenase (G-6-PD), 171-172
Glyburide, 55, 61, 83, 90, 119-20, 123, 159, 176, 236, 255, 278
Glycerin,120, 134, 236, 255, 277
Glycogen storage disease, 118, 121, 277
Glycopyrrolate, 55, 61, 83, 90
Glycosuria, 31, 168-9
Glycosylated Hemoglobin, (A1C) 154-5, 161-2, 166, 168, 173-6
Gold, 194
Goodpasture's syndrome, 235
Goserelin, 55, 83, 157, 277
Gout, 277
Granisetron, 55, 83
Granulocyte colonizing factor, 120, 194
Granulomatous diseases, 109, 231
Graves' disease, 265, 271, 272, 274
Griseofulvin, 55, 61, 83, 90, 96, 134, 236, 239
Growth hormone, 157, 210, 228, 254, 266
Guanabenz, 120
Guanethidine, 55, 61, 83, 90, 96, 113, 159, 254
Guar, 159
Hairy-cell-leukemia, 296
Haloperidol, 55, 61, 83, 90, 120, 127, 158-9, 198, 255
Halothane, 90
Hashimoto's thyroiditis, 265, 271
HDL, 23, 66-9, 100, 114-121, 262
Head & neck cancer, 103
Heat stroke, 81, 192
Heavy-metal poisoning, 138, 235
Hematocrit, (HCT) , 22, 33, 156, 177-9, 181, 240-3, 245
Hematoma, 88
Hematuria, 189

Hemochromatosis, 141, 143, 156, 166, 187-90
Hemodialysis, 69, 70, 143, 175
Hemoglobin, (HGB), 51, 178, 180-2, 186-7, 240-3, 245, 299
Hemoglobinuria, 235
Hemolysis, 39-41, 87, 172, 182, 215, 229, 242-3, 289
Hemolytic anemia, 38, 47, 80, 88, 118, 141, 143, 144, 148, 149, 172, 175,
    178, 188, 190, 191, 193, 210, 242, 243, 245, 289
Hemolytic jaundice, 88
Hemophilia, 127
Hemorrhage, 95, 126, 127, 131, 143, 178, 182, 215, 227, 245
Hemosiderosis, 141-143, 187, 189, 190
Heparin, 55, 56, 83, 119, 120, 215, 216, 239, 266, 278, 295
Hepatic coma, 63, 172
Hepatic encephalopathy, 63
Hepatic ischemia, 53
Hepatic metastasis, 81
Hepatitis A vaccine, 55, 61, 83, 90, 236
Hepatitis B vaccine, 55, 61, 83, 90
Hepatitis, 53, 80, 87, 88, 274
Hepatobiliary disease, 290
Hepatoma, 121, 149
Hetastarch, 134
HHH syndrome, 64
High altitudes, 177-8, 181, 244
Histrelin, 170
HIV, 269
HMG CoA-reductase inhibitors, 120, 278
Hodgkin's disease, 59, 103, 108, 139, 146, 223
Homocysteine, (Hcy) 45-7, 50-1, 100, 183-5, 200, 247, 283
Homocystinuria, 184-5
High Sensitivity CRP, (hs-CRP), 17, 98-100
Hydralazine, 55, 61, 83, 90, 96, 105, 120, 134, 140, 158-9, 194, 236, 284
Hydrochlorothiazide 55, 60, 64, 83, 90, 96, 105, 110, 113, 134, 158, 170,
    176, 198, 210, 217, 219, 255, 257, 277
Hydrocortisone, 77, 113, 123, 127, 150, 219, 254, 257, 266, 275
Hydroflumethiazide, 55, 61, 64, 83, 90, 96, 113, 158, 198, 255, 257
Hydroquinone, 170
Hydroxychloroquine, 120, 134, 140, 278
Hydroxyurea, 90-1, 96, 134, 194, 278
Hyperaldosteronism, 197, 215, 251, 253
Hyperammonemia, 64
Hypercalcemia, 102-3, 108, 197, 205, 207, 209
Hyperchloremia, 112
Hypercholesterolemia, 71, 230
Hyperfibrinogenemia, 138
Hyperglycemia, 152, 173-5, 205, 215, 254
Hyperinsulinism, 209
Hyperlipidemia, 118, 166, 277
Hyperlipoproteinemia, 70-1
Hypermagnesemia 195-7
Hypernatremia, 112, 205, 207, 251-2

Hyperornithinemia, 64
Hyperosmolar nonketotic hyperglycemia, 205
Hyperparathyroidism, 59, 101-4, 108, 112, 209, 287
Hyperphosphatasia, 59
Hyperproteinemia, 205, 271, 274
Hypersplenism, 295
Hypertension, 63-4, 100, 118, 182, 202, 234-5, 262, 277
Hyperthermia, 126-7, 193
Hyperthyroidism, 56, 70, 104, 118, 121, 123, 133, 137-8, 143, 149, 156, 163, 165-6, 172, 178, 190, 221, 227, 229, 235, 241, 260-77, 296
Hypertonic dehydration, 32-3
Hypertonic overhydration, 34-5
Hypertriglyceridemia, 69, 121, 155, 205, 253, 262
Hyperventilation, 78, 104, 112
Hypoalbuminemia, 34, 43, 103-4
Hypoaldosteronism, 215
Hypocalcemia, 103, 108, 196, 209, 287
Hypochloremia, 76, 111-2
Hypochromic anemia, 42, 186, 242
Hypocitrullinuria, 64
Hypofibrinogenemia, 138
Hypoglycemia, 152, 156, 165, 167
Hypokalemia, 63, 76, 111-2, 126-7, 196, 207, 211-215
Hyponatremia, 33, 111-2, 205, 251-3
Hypoparathyroidism, 103-104, 108, 166, 197, 210, 288
Hypophosphatemia, 59, 107, 208-9, 287
Hypopituitarism, 123, 156, 163, 166, 205, 264
Hypoproteinemia, 190, 233, 270
Hypotension, 111, 193, 196, 214
Hypothalamic failure, 267, 271-2, 274
Hypothermia, 126-7, 210
Hypothyroidism, 126-7, 137-8, 149, 156, 163, 166, 182, 193, 197, 209, 248-9, 254, 256, 261-75
Hypotonic dehydration, 32-3
Hypotonic overhydration, 34-5
Ibandronate, 110, 119
Ibuprofen, 55, 61, 83, 85, 90, 96, 119, 134-5, 194, 236-7, 257
Idarubicin, 55, 61, 83, 90, 96, 134
Ifosfamide, 55, 61, 83, 96, 170, 236, 257
Ileal resection, 49, 241
Ileus, 253
Imatinib, 55, 83, 134, 217
Imipenem/cilastin, 55, 61, 83
Imipramine, 55, 61, 62, 83, 90, 92, 96, 119, 134, 158, 160, 194
Immune globin, 96, 134
Indapamide, 90, 119, 158, 176, 217, 237
Indinavir, 55, 83, 90, 158
Indomethacin, 55, 61, 70, 83, 90, 92, 96, 120, 124, 134, 140, 158, 160, 170, 179, 182, 215, 219, 236, 255, 257, 278

Infection, 16-7, 31, 35, 38, 42, 53, 63-4, 98-100, 118, 121, 139, 142, 146, 153, 165-6, 168, 171-2, 187-9, 215, 223, 227, 230-2, 235, 246, 269, 281, 291-7
Infectious mononucleosis, 53, 59, 80, 81, 193, 296
Inflammation/ Inflammatory response, 16-7, 34, 42, 52, 80, 87-8, 92, 99-100, 118, 142, 145, 187, 220-226, 231, 292, 295, 299
Inflammatory bowel disease, 189, 286, 288
Inflammatory joint disease, 70, 121
Infliximab, 55, 83
Insulin, 105, 120, 122, 123, 127, 151-6, 160-6, 168, 170, 175-6, 198, 209, 210, 217, 228, 257, 275, 278
Insulinoma, 156, 163
Interferon, 55, 57, 61, 70, 83, 90, 105, 109, 123, 135, 158, 160, 194, 198, 236, 266, 275, 277
Interleukin, 38, 55, 61, 83, 90, 96, 98, 123, 127, 134, 194
International Normal Ratio, (INR), 238-9
Intestinal ischemia, 60, 126, 193
Intestinal resection, 149
Intestinal worm infestation, 286
Intravascular hemolysis, 242
Intrinsic factor (IF), 48-50, 241, 247-249, 285
Iodine deficiency, 271-2, 274
Ion exchange resins, 65, 113, 271
Irbesartan, 96, 134
Irinotecan, 61, 90, 158
Iron, serum (Fe), 51, 143, 186-90
Iron Deficiency Anemia, 41-2, 141-3, 181, 186-190, 228, 230, 240-3
Iron Dextran, 90, 105
Iron malabsorption, 240
Iron poisoning, 188-9
Ischemic coronary disease, 69
Islet cell carcinoma, 156
Isocarboxazid, 160
Isoniazid, (INH), 90, 92, 105, 120, 150, 158, 160, 170, 210, 216, 236, 284, 288
Isoproterenol, 158
Isosorbide dinitrate, 55, 83, 120, 255
Isotonic dehydration, 32-3
Isotonic overhydration, 34-5
Isotretinoin, 55, 70, 83, 90, 91, 119, 120, 127, 134, 140, 158, 194, 236, 272, 273, 275, 277
Isradipine, 55, 61, 83, 90, 120
Itraconazole, 55, 61, 83, 90, 127, 194, 217, 255, 277
Jaundice, 87-8
Jejunal bypass procedure, 149
Kanamycin, 55, 61, 65, 83, 90, 96, 120, 134, 146, 236
Ketamine, 55, 61, 83
Ketoconazole, 55, 61, 70, 83, 90, 105, 110, 120, 124, 216, 219, 255, 278
Ketoprofen, 55, 57, 61, 83, 85, 90, 96, 131, 134-5, 137, 158, 217, 254, 255
Ketorolac, 55, 61, 83, 90, 96, 134, 216, 236, 255, 257
Ketosis, 205

Kidney disease, 38, 93-4, 108-9, 129-30, 168, 221, 223, 234-5
Kostmann's syndrome, 295
Labetalol, 55, 61, 83, 90, 96, 124, 127, 134, 158, 216, 277
Lactic dehydrogenase (LDH),53, 59, 79, 80, 88, 126, 191-194, 279
Lactobacillus acidophilus, 65
Lactose, 158
Lactulose, 65, 134
Lamivudine, 90, 127
Lamotrigine, 55, 61, 83, 90, 134, 146
Lansoprazole, 90, 119, 120, 134, 158, 160, 236
Laronidase, 90
Laxatives, 105, 113, 217, 249, 255
LDL, 23, 67-9, 114-121, 183, 262, 276
Lead poisoning, 176, 189, 241
Leflunomide, 55, 61, 83, 105, 140
Leukemia, 103, 109, 137, 144, 149, 178, 182, 189, 193, 235, 246, 286, 295-7
Leuprolide, 96, 105, 134, 158, 160
Levalbuterol, 158, 217
Levamisole, 55, 83, 90, 127
Levarterenol, 157, 219, 257
Levodopa, 55, 61, 65, 83, 90, 96, 97, 105, 124, 134, 150, 158, 160, 170, 194, 217, 219, 257, 278
Levofloxacin, 158, 160
Levonorgestrel, 70, 120, 158, 278
Levorphanol, 96
Levothyroxine, 56, 61, 70, 83, 120, 266, 271-5, 277-8
Licorice, 215, 219
Lidocaine, 127, 134
Lincomycin, 56, 61, 83, 90, 120, 150
Liothyronine, 158
Lipomul, 236
Lipoprotein (a), 66-71
Lisinopril, 56, 61, 70, 83, 90, 96, 119, 120, 134, 158, 160, 176, 216, 255
Lithium, 61, 96, 105, 109-10, 113, 119, 123-4, 127, 134, 158, 170, 198, 210, 216-7, 219, 236, 255, 257, 266, 272-3, 275
Liver cancer/metastasis, 59, 88, 92, 103
Liver disease, 63, 71, 118, 121, 123, 133, 141-6, 148-9, 155-6, 163, 166-7, 188-90, 204, 215, 221, 226, 229, 240, 249, 269, 286, 288
Lomefloxacin, 56, 61, 83, 90, 96, 140, 160, 217
Loop diuretics,34, 77-8, 113, 198
Loperamide, 158
Loracarbef, 56, 61, 83, 96, 134
Loratadine, 56, 61, 83
Losartan, 56, 70, 83, 90, 96, 120, 134, 257
Lovastatin, 56, 61, 69, 70, 83, 90, 127, 134, 146, 176, 216, 266, 278
Loxapine, 56, 83, 90, 128
Lugol's iodine, 90
Lung cancer, 59, 103, 207
Lupus erythematosus, 139, 215, 229, 235, 296
Lymphocytes, 291-297

Lymphoma, 109, 139, 193
Macroalbuminuria, 234
Macrocytic anemia, 38-9, 44-51, 141-4, 147-9, 241-3
Macroglobulinemia, 138, 230-1
Mafenide, 219
Magnesium, 28, 59, 63, 104, 105, 109-110, 124, 195-8, 209, 213
Malabsorption, 41, 47, 49-50, 103-4, 118, 121, 148-9, 197, 155, 163, 165-6, 197, 208, 214, 226, 238-40, 248-9, 254, 256, 260, 277, 280, 282-6, 288-90, 298
Malaria, 246
Maldigestion, 163
Malnutrition, 35, 53, 59, 70-1, 95, 103, 118, 121, 133, 142, 145-6, 148, 163, 179, 182, 185, 188, 190, 197, 210, 221, 223, 229-30, 268-70, 274, 277, 281-4, 299
Mannitol, 109, 113, 134, 210, 216, 254, 255, 257
MAO inhibitors, 56, 61, 65, 83, 90, 120, 160
Maple syrup urine disease, 156
Maprotiline, 56, 83, 158, 160
Mean corpuscular hemoglobin concentration(MCHC), 23, 178-81, 240-3
Mean Corpuscular Hemoglobin(MCH), 23, 55, 178, 181, 240-3
Mean Corpuscular Volume(MCV), 23, 38-40, 47-51, 178, 181, 240-5
Mechlorethamine, 56, 61, 83
Meclofenamate, 56, 61, 83, 96, 134
Medroxyprogesterone, 56, 61, 83, 90, 119-20, 124, 146, 158, 198, 210, 278
Mefenamic acid, 56, 83, 90, 96, 135, 158, 236
Mefloquine, 56, 83
Megaloblastic anemia, 40-1, 43, 50-1, 143-4, 147-9, 172, 182-3, 188, 191, 193, 240, 245
Megestrol, 124, 158, 160
Melphalan, 56, 61, 83, 90, 96
Mental retardation, 118, 271
Mepazine, 119
Meperidine, 56, 83, 90, 128, 158, 194
Meprobamate, 56, 61, 83, 90, 119
Mercaptopurine, 56, 61, 83, 90, 158
Mercurial diuretics, 77
Meropenem, 56, 61, 83, 90, 96, 135
Mesalamine, 56, 61, 83, 90, 96, 124, 135, 194, 236
Mesoridazine, 90
Mestranol, 110, 211, 269, 272, 273, 275, 284
Metabolic acidosis 73-8, 104, 112, 215
Metabolic alkalosis 73-77, 109, 111-2, 219
Metabolic syndrome, 100, 120
Metaxalone, 56, 61, 83, 90, 150, 236
Metformin, 120, 150, 160, 176, 189, 249, 278, 286
Methacholine, 90, 150
Methadone, 123, 269, 272-3, 275
Methandrostenolone, 158
Methazolamide, 109, 217
Methenamine, 56, 83, 150, 236

Methicillin, 77, 96, 105, 135, 189, 210, 216, 236
Methimazole, 56, 61, 83, 90, 119, 144, 158, 189, 203, 216, 266, 272-3, 275, 278
Methotrexate, 47, 56, 61, 83, 90, 96, 131, 135, 137, 140, 148, 150, 185, 189, 194, 210
Methoxsalen, 56, 61, 83, 90
Methsuximide, 90, 96
Methyclothiazide, 70, 90, 96, 105, 109, 110, 113, 119, 158, 170, 198, 217, 219, 254, 255, 257, 277
Methyl malonic acid(MMA), 49-51, 199-200
Methyldopa, 56, 61, 83, 90, 92, 96, 113, 120, 131, 135, 137, 140, 158, 160, 179, 182, 189, 194, 239, 254, 277
Methylene blue, 90, 172
Methylphenidate, 56, 83, 90
Methylprednisolone, 124, 135, 158, 217, 255, 257
Methyltestosterone, 56, 61, 83, 90, 105, 113, 119, 160, 210, 216, 254, 269
Methysergide, 96, 140
Metoclopramide, 56, 61, 83, 90, 105, 123, 217, 266
Metolazone, 56, 61, 83, 90, 96, 105, 110, 113, 158, 170, 198, 217, 219, 255, 257, 260
Metoprolol, 56, 61, 70, 83, 96, 120, 135, 158, 160, 194, 216, 257, 275, 277
Metronidazole, 85, 120, 158, 160, 194
Mexiletine, 56, 83
Micardis, 96, 135, 216
Miconazole, 119, 255, 277
Microcytic anemia, 39, 241-3
Midazolam, 124, 160
Miglitol, 160
Milk-alkali syndrome, 59, 104, 107, 109, 210
Milrinone, 217
Minocycline, 56, 61, 83, 90, 96, 140, 210
Mirtazapine, 56, 61, 83, 90, 119, 158, 170, 277
Misoprostol, 61, 96, 140, 170
Mithramycin, 194
Mitomycin, 56, 83, 90, 96, 135, 236
Mitotane, 236, 275
Mitoxantrone, 56, 61, 83, 90, 96, 135
Moexipril, 56, 61, 83, 97, 135, 216
Molindone, 56, 61, 83, 90, 97, 158
Monocytes, 291-297
Montelukast, 56, 83
Moricizine, 56, 83, 90, 217
Morphine, 56, 61, 63, 83, 90, 124, 128, 158, 194, 203, 255, 266
Moxalactam, 56, 61, 83, 90, 97, 135, 217, 236
Multiple myeloma, 103, 109, 112, 121, 139, 146, 178, 182, 230-1, 234, 296
Multiple organ failure, 104
Muromonab-CD3, 56, 83
Muscular dystrophy, 81, 126, 127, 133, 137, 192
Mushroom poisoning, 80
Mycophenolate, 56, 61, 83, 105, 119, 135, 158, 160, 194, 211, 216, 217, 236
Myelodysplastic syndromes, 246

Myelofibrosis, 46, 149, 295
Myeloproliferative disease, 118, 121, 286, 296
Myocardial infarction(MI), 79, 95, 118, 126, 146
Myocarditis, 126, 127, 279
Myoglobinuria, 236
Myopathy, 81
Myositis, 54, 126
Myxedema, 165, 166, 271, 272, 274
Nabumetone, 56, 61, 83, 90, 92, 97, 158, 217, 236
Nadolol, 160, 277
Nafarelin, 56, 61, 83, 119, 210, 277
Nafcillin, 56, 83, 170, 236
Nalidixic acid, 56, 61, 83, 90, 97, 135, 158, 170, 172
Naltrexone, 56, 61, 83, 85, 194
Nandrolone, 56, 61, 83, 105, 110, 119, 120, 131, 135, 137, 160, 269, 277
Naphthalene, 236
Naproxen, 56, 61, 83, 90, 97, 119, 135, 158, 170, 210, 216-7, 236, 257, 275
Natriuretic peptides (ANP, BNP, NT-pro-BNP), 201-3
Necrosis, 53, 81, 95, 123, 130-3, 145, 189, 193, 205, 207, 231, 292, 295
Nefazodone, 56, 83, 119, 160, 194
Nelfinavir, 56, 61, 83, 128, 158, 160, 194
Neomycin, 65, 70, 71, 97, 110, 120, 135, 198, 217, 236, 239, 249, 286
Neostigmine, 113
Nephritis, 112, 131, 133, 139, 188, 215, 235, 256
Nephrosis, 118, 139, 143, 188
Nephrotic syndrome, 68-70, 84, 95, 118, 121, 131, 143, 146, 189, 223, 227, 229, 231, 233-5, 254, 257, 277, 288
Netilmicin, 56, 61, 83, 90, 97, 135, 216, 236, 275
Neutrophils, 291-7
Nevirapine, 56, 83, 90
Niacin, 56, 61, 69, 70, 71, 83, 90, 100, 120, 128, 158, 160, 170, 176, 211, 219, 257, 278, 283
Niacinamide, 56, 61, 83, 90, 120, 158, 219, 257
Nicardipine, 56, 61, 83, 90, 135, 176, 211, 255, 278
Nicotine, 166
Nicotinic acid, 70, 90, 120, 158, 170, 176, 278
Nifedipine, 56, 61, 70, 83, 97, 120, 124, 128, 135, 158, 160, 194, 203, 210, 216-7, 237, 255, 257, 266, 278
Nilutamide, 56, 61, 83, 97, 135, 158, 217
Nisoldipine, 56, 69, 83, 97, 105, 128, 135, 158, 176, 217, 255, 278
Nitazoxanide, 56, 83, 135
Nitisinone, 56, 83
Nitrofurantoin, 56, 61, 77, 83, 90, 97, 131, 135, 137, 150, 158, 170, 172, 194, 210, 254-5
Nitrous oxide, 124, 185
Nizatidine, 56, 61, 83, 90
Non-Hodgkin's disease, 103
Nonspherocytic anemia, 172
Non-steroidal anti-inflammatory drugs (NSAID), 135, 140, 237, 255
Norethandrolone, 56, 61, 83, 90, 92, 119, 146, 269
Norethindrone, 62, 90, 124, 158, 160, 269, 272-3, 278

Norfloxacin, 56, 61, 83, 97, 119, 135, 158, 160, 170, 194, 216, 237, 277
Norplant, 119, 120
Nortriptyline, 56, 61, 83, 90, 158, 160
Novobiocin, 90
Obesity, 77, 118, 121, 123, 154, 156, 276
Obstruction of urinary tract, 131
Obstructive jaundice 54, 59
Octreotide, 56, 61, 83, 90, 110, 123, 158, 160, 249, 257, 266, 272-3, 286
Ofloxacin, 56, 61, 84, 90, 97, 119, 135, 140, 158, 160, 170, 194, 216, 237, 277
Olanzapine, 128, 158, 255
Oleandomycin, 56, 61, 84, 90
Oliguria, 197, 257
Olmesartan, 119, 277
Olsalazine, 56, 61, 84, 97, 135, 237
Omeprazole, 56, 61, 84, 90, 170, 249, 255, 257, 286
Ondansetron, 56, 84, 217
Open heart surgery, 126
Opiates, 123, 275
Oral contraceptives, 62, 69, 70, 84, 90, 92, 100, 105, 110, 119-21, 123, 128, 140, 144, 146, 150, 158, 185, 189-90, 198, 203, 210-1, 219, 223, 228, 239, 249, 254, 257, 269, 272-3, 275, 277, 286
Orlistat, 120
Osmolality, 23, 33, 35, 111, 204-7, 250-2, 258
Osmotic dilution, 254
Osmotic diuresis, 253
Osmotic hyperglycemia, 215
Osteogenic sarcoma, 59
Osteomalacia, 60, 104, 209, 287
Osteomyelitis, 44
Osteoporosis, 109, 185, 262
Ovarian failure, 269
Overhydration, 29-34, 38, 95, 112, 178, 181, 189, 204-5, 213, 223, 226
Oxacillin, 56, 61, 84, 90, 97, 135, 194, 237, 272, 273
Oxaliplatin, 90
Oxandrolone, 120, 146, 160, 278
Oxaprozin, 56, 61, 84, 97, 135, 194, 237
Oxazepam, 56, 61, 84, 90, 124, 158
Oxymetholone, 56, 61, 84, 90, 105, 119, 120, 131, 137, 146, 160, 189, 269
Oxytetracycline, 97, 160, 170
Paget's disease, 60, 104, 109
Palivizumab, 56, 84
Palonosetron, 158, 216
Pamidronate, 62, 97, 105, 110, 135, 198, 211, 217
Pancreatic cancer 59, 103, 109, 121, 166
Pancreatitis, 54, 80, 103, 104, 156, 165-6, 193, 197, 277, 290
Pancreozymin, 158
Panhypopituitarism, 205
Papaverine, 56, 61, 84, 90
Paracentesis, 63
Paraldehyde, 77, 158, 237

Paramethadione, 237
Paramethasone, 257
Parasites, 241, 296
Parathyroid hormone (PTH), 101, 104, 108, 208-9, 287-8
Pargyline, 56, 61, 84, 90, 97, 160
Paromomycin, 97, 135, 237
Paroxetine, 56, 61, 84, 90, 97, 105, 119, 128, 158, 160, 194, 210, 216-7, 255
PCO2, 72-8
Pegaptanib, 158
Pegaspargase, 56, 62, 65, 84, 90, 97, 135, 146, 158, 160
Pegfilgrastim, 194
Peginterferon, 266
Pemoline, 56, 84, 90, 194
Penicillamine, 56, 62, 84, 85, 90, 97, 119, 128, 135, 140, 160, 185, 194, 216, 237, 275, 284
Penicillin, 90, 92, 97, 128, 135, 150, 170, 179, 182, 216, 217, 219, 237, 254
Pentamidine, 56, 84, 97, 105, 120, 135, 150, 158, 160, 198, 216
Pentostatin, 97, 105, 255
Pentoxifylline, 56, 84, 90, 146, 278
Pergolide, 119, 158, 160, 189, 217
Pericarditis, 79
Perindopril, 120, 158, 160, 216, 237, 277
Peripheral edema, 252, 254, 260
Peripheral vascular disease, 146, 185
Pernicious anemia, 41, 43-4, 46-51, 59, 88, 118, 139, 143-4, 148-9, 172, 181, 188-90, 193, 200, 241, 245, 247-9, 285-6
Perphenazine, 56, 62, 84, 90, 92, 158, 160, 170, 269
Phenacetin, 172
Phenazopyridine, 56, 62, 84, 90, 92, 97, 135, 158, 160, 170, 172, 228, 237
Phenelzine, 56, 84, 90, 128, 158, 254
Phenformin hydrochloride, 77
Phenobarbital, 56, 62, 69, 70, 84, 90, 105, 110, 119, 124, 150, 170, 272-3, 275, 288
Phenolphthalein, 237
Phenothiazine, 56-7, 62, 84, 90, 92, 97, 119, 121, 128, 158, 170, 211, 269, 275
Phenoxybenzamine, 255
Phentolamine, 160
Phenylbutazone, 56, 84
Phenylephrine, 158
Phenytoin, 56, 62, 69, 70, 84, 90, 105, 110, 124, 128, 150, 158, 170, 185, 211, 266, 269, 271-3, 275, 288
Pheochromocytoma, 156, 163-4, 167, 176
Phosphate, (PO4), 23, 107, 171-2, 208-10
Phosphorus, 56, 62, 84, 90, 97, 135, 146, 160, 208-11, 237
Phospho-soda, 210
Pimozide, 255
Pindolol, 56, 62, 84, 85, 92, 119, 120, 128, 158, 194, 210, 216, 277, 278
Pioglitazone, 56, 84, 128, 160
Piperacillin, 56, 62, 84, 91, 97, 135, 170, 194, 217, 237

Piroxicam, 56, 62, 84, 91, 97, 135, 158, 160, 216, 237
Pituitary adenoma, 156
Pituitary insufficiency, 271-2, 274
Pleural effusion, 252, 253
Plicamycin, 97, 105, 110, 135, 194, 211, 217, 237
Plummer's disease, 271-2, 274
Pneumonia, 139, 146, 192
Poliomyelitis, 133
Polycystic disease, 234
Polycythemia vera, 135, 178, 181, 189, 190, 286
Polymyalgia rheumatica, 138-9
Polymyositis, 81, 126, 127, 137
Polymyxin B, 237
Polystyrene sulfonate, 105, 217, 254
Polythiazide, 56, 62, 84, 91, 105, 110, 113, 119, 158, 170, 217, 255, 257, 277
Porphyria, 70, 112, 121, 187, 269
Post gastrectomy, 167
Posthemorrhagic anemias, 242-3
Postsplenectomy, 246
Potassium chloride 216
Potassium iodine, 266, 275
Potassium, 23, 28, 34, 65, 111-2, 195, 197, 209, 212-19
Pralidoxime, 56, 84, 255
Pramipexole, 128
Pravastatin, 56, 69, 70, 84, 119, 120, 124, 128, 146, 158, 176, 255, 278
Prazosin, 56, 70, 84, 91, 120, 128, 158, 160, 203, 266, 277, 278
Pre- Eclampsia , 234, 236
Prealbumin (PAB), 14, 17, 35, 98, 220-32, 280, 282, 299
Prednisolone, 69, 70, 110, 119, 120, 123, 124, 140, 198, 217, 219, 223, 228, 254, 277-8
Prednisone, 62, 85, 92, 105, 113, 123, 124, 128, 131, 135, 137, 140, 146, 158, 160, 217, 254, 266, 269, 275, 296
Pregabalin, 237
Pregnancy, 58-9, 69-70, 77-80, 95, 109, 118, 130, 139, 146, 148-9, 155-6, 169, 175, 178, 188-90, 197, 223, 227, 246, 256, 258, 269-70, 274, 277, 286
Pressure ulcers, 14, 227
Primaquine, 91, 172
Primidone, 150
Probenecid, 56, 62, 84, 91, 97, 158, 160, 170, 237
Probucol, 70, 105, 120, 128, 278
Procainamide, 56, 62, 84, 91, 128,140, 194, 216
Procarbazine, 91
Prochlorperazine, 56, 62, 84, 91, 119
Progesterone, 85, 91, 105, 120, 160, 198, 228, 254, 257, 269
Promazine, 91, 119, 237
Promethazine, 62, 91, 128, 160
Propafenone, 56, 62, 84, 91, 97, 135, 140, 158, 255
Propoxyphene, 56, 62, 84, 91, 160, 194
Propranolol, 56, 84, 97, 105, 119, 128, 135, 158, 160, 176, 194, 216, 257, 266, 269, 271, 273, 275, 277

Propylthiouracil, 56, 62, 84, 91, 97, 158, 194, 239, 271, 273, 275
Prostate cancer 109, 121
Prosthetic valves, 178, 182
Protein, Serum, 35-37, 220-32
Protein, Urine, 233-7
Prothrombin time (PT), 238-9
Protriptyline, 62, 158, 160
Psyllium, 70, 120, 278
Pulmonary edema, 77-8
Pulmonary emboli, 77-80, 126, 192
Pulmonary infarction, 99, 100, 125, 126, 192
Pyelonephritis, 95, 131, 133, 205, 207, 219, 235
Pyrazinamide, 56, 62, 84, 91, 146, 189
Pyridoxal phosphate (PLP), 283
Pyrimethamine, 56, 62, 84, 150
Quazepam, 56, 62, 84, 91, 97, 135
Quinapril, 57, 62, 84, 91, 97, 110, 131, 135, 137, 158, 160, 216, 237
Quinethazone, 62, 91, 97, 158, 170, 217, 219, 255, 257
Quinidine, 57, 62, 84, 91, 128, 140, 172, 194, 239
Quinine, 91, 97, 160, 237, 239, 295
Quinupristin, 91, 194, 216
Radiation therapy (Radiographic agents),91, 97, 135, 170, 237, 246, 266, 271, 273, 275, 292, 295, 296
Radioactive iodine, 70, 119, 277
Raloxifene, 70, 105, 120, 146, 211, 269
Ramipril, 57, 62, 84, 91, 97, 120, 135, 158, 160, 176, 203, 216, 219, 237, 254, 255, 257
Ranitidine, 57, 62, 84, 91, 123, 124, 135, 237, 249, 272, 273, 275, 286
Reactive hypoglycemia, 156, 165, 167
Red blood cell distribution width (RDW), 40, 42, 178, 181, 240-3
Red blood cell indicies 240-3
Refeeding, 208-10, 220, 222, 226
Regional enteritis, 249, 299
Reiter's syndrome, 100
Renal artery stenosis, 215
Renal cell cancer, 103, 144
Renal dialysis, 69, 70, 80, 143, 175, 279
Renal disease, 29, 43, 73, 118, 121, 130, 139, 184, 197, 221, 258
Renal failure, 15, 44, 64, 68-9, 71, 76-8, 80, 95, 101, 103-4, 127, 138-9, 141, 149, 156, 163, 165-6, 175, 185, 196, 200, 205-6, 209, 214, 219, 256, 271, 275, 279, 288, 298
Renal transplant, 101, 104, 193, 202, 215, 235, 293
Renal tubular acidosis, 109, 112, 214, 219
Renal tubular necrosis 205, 207
Renal vein thrombosis, 235
Repaglinide, 160
Resection of terminal ileum, 286
Reserpine, 91, 158, 170, 275
Respiratory acidosis 74-7, 112
Respiratory alkalosis, 73-77, 112, 210, 215
Reteplase, 146

Reticular agenesis, 295
Reticulocyte count, 40, 42, 47, 51, 244-6
Retinol binding protein (RBP), 220-32, 282
Reye's syndrome, 63-4, 70, 81, 121, 126-7
Rhabdomyolysis, 103, 126-7, 133, 210, 279
Rheumatic carditis, 79
Rheumatic fever, 44, 98, 100, 139, 295
Rheumatoid arthritis 44, 60, 98, 100, 139, 146, 182, 295
Rickets, 59, 103, 287-8
Rickets, 59, 103, 287-8
Rifampin, 57, 62, 84, 85, 91, 97, 124, 150, 158, 179, 182, 210, 237, 249, 266, 286, 288
Riluzole, 57, 62, 84, 91, 105, 119, 158, 194, 217, 255
Risedronate, 110, 210, 216
Risperidone, 57, 62, 84, 97, 128, 135, 158, 189, 210, 217, 255, 277
Ritodrine, 170, 217
Ritonavir, 57, 84, 97, 119, 128, 158, 278
Rosiglitazone, 57, 84, 119, 160
Rotor's syndrome, 88, 92
Rubella, 296
Salicylate, 77, 78, 91, 112, 223
Salsalate, 135, 237, 275
Salt-losing nephritis, 112, 256
Saquinavir, 57, 84, 91, 158, 160
Sarcoidosis, 59, 103, 104, 109, 182, 209, 231
Sargramostim, 57, 62, 84, 91, 97, 105, 119, 135, 158
Schilling test, 50, 149, 247-9, 286
Scleroderma, 249
Scurvy, 59
Secobarbital, 170
Secretin, 257,
Seizures, 126, 193, 204-5, 251, 283
Selegiline, 160
Semustine, 57, 84, 97
Sepsis, 88, 118, 210, 221, 296, 298
Sertraline, 255
Severe shock syndrome, 126
Sevoflurane, 135, 170, 237
Shock, 20, 32, 54, 74, 76-7, 81, 94, 104, 126-7, 129-30, 133, 178, 193, 205, 207, 260
Shwachman-Diamond syndrome, 295
SIADH, 95, 112, 197, 205, 207, 252, 254, 256
Sibutramine, 57, 84, 194
Sickle cell anemia, 88, 138, 182, 189-91, 242-3, 246, 284
Sideroblastic anemia 118, 143, 144, 188
Sildenafil, 57, 62, 84, 158, 160, 254
Silver, 97, 237
Simvastatin, 57, 69-70, 84-5, 120, 128, 146, 160, 278
Sirolimus, 105, 119, 128, 135, 198, 210-1, 216, 255
Skeletal muscle trauma, 81
Small bowel diverticula, 249

Smoking, 63, 67, 100, 121, 146, 153, 156, 166-7, 184, 276
Sodium Bicarbonate, 198, 217, 237, 254, 255
Sodium oxybate, 57, 84, 110, 119, 135, 158, 237
Sodium sulfate, 254
Sodium, 23, 28, 32-5, 108, 111-2, 155, 195, 197, 201, 212-4, 224, 250-9
Somatostatin, 158, 160, 255, 266, 275
Somatropin, 170, 216
Somogyi response, 167
Sorbitan, 91
Sotalol, 119, 278
Sparfloxacin, 57, 84
Specific Gravity, Urine, 258
Spectinomycin, 57, 62, 84, 97
Spherocytosis, 138, 243
Spironolactone, 91, 97, 105, 110, 119, 120, 123, 135, 158, 216, 217, 255, 257, 278
Splenectomy, 176, 246, 292
Splenomegaly, 182, 282
Sprue, 47, 104, 149, 166, 227, 241, 281-2, 288, 299
St. John's wort, 160
Stanozolol, 57, 62, 70, 71, 84, 91, 269, 275, 278
Starvation, 77, 78, 94, 95, 155, 219, 225, 267
Statins, 100, 120
Stavudine, 57, 84, 91
Streptokinase, 57, 62, 84, 97, 120, 135, 146, 194, 237
Streptomycin, 57, 84, 91, 97, 135, 158, 170
Streptozocin, 57, 84, 105, 135, 158, 194, 217, 219
Stress, 16, 95, 118, 122, 123, 125, 142, 151-3, 156, 163, 166-9, 171, 174, 176, 187, 189, 215, 220, 222-6, 231, 235, 269, 292, 294-8
Struma ovarii, 271-2, 275
Subarachnoid hemorrhage, 126-7
Succinylcholine, 216
Sucralfate, 211
Sulfacetamide, 91
Sulfadiazine, 57, 62, 84, 91, 119, 237
Sulfamethizole, 91
Sulfamethoxazole, 57, 62, 84, 91, 97, 128, 135, 140, 150, 160, 194, 216, 219, 237
Sulfasalazine, 57, 62, 84, 91, 97, 135, 140, 150, 194, 237
Sulfinpyrazone, 91
Sulfisoxazole, 57, 62, 84, 91, 92, 97, 135, 146, 150, 158, 160, 194, 237
Sulfonamide, 92, 119, 121, 170, 172, 179, 182, 239, 295
Sulfonylureas, 57, 62, 84, 91, 255, 275
Sulindac, 57, 62, 84, 91, 97, 135, 158, 194, 216, 237
Sumatriptan, 57, 84, 124, 158, 160, 266
Suprofen, 97, 135, 237
Syphilis, 139
Tacrine, 57, 84, 91, 158, 170
Tacrolimus, 57, 62, 70, 84, 91, 97, 105, 120, 135, 158, 198, 210, 211, 216, 217, 237, 255
Tadalafil, 57, 84

Tamoxifen, 57, 62, 84, 91, 105, 119-20, 140, 185, 266, 269, 271, 273, 275, 278
Tangier's disease, 69, 70
Tegaserod, 57, 84, 237
Telithromycin, 91
Temporal arteritis, 138-9
Tenofovir, 278
Terazosin, 120, 135, 160, 176, 278
Terbinafine, 57, 62, 84, 91
Terbutaline, 57, 84, 158, 160, 217, 275
Testicular cancer , 193
Testosterone, 91, 119, 189, 269
Tetracycline, 57, 62, 65, 77, 84, 91, 97, 105, 119, 120, 135, 150, 158, 160, 170, 210, 217, 237, 254, 257
Thalassemia, 143-4, 176, 182, 188, 190, 240-1, 243
Thallium, 97, 237
Theophylline, 91-2, 105, 119, 140, 144, 158, 170, 185, 198, 210-1, 217, 237, 255, 275, 288
Thiabendazole, 57, 62, 84, 91, 119, 158, 160, 237
Thiamin, 259-60
Thiazide Diuretics, 77, 172
Thiethylperazine, 57, 62, 84, 91
Thiocyanate, 57, 84
Thioguanine, 57, 62, 84, 91
Thiopental, 57, 62, 84, 91
Thioridazine, 57, 62, 84, 91-2
Thiothixene, 57, 62, 84, 91, 158, 170
Thiouracil, 57, 62, 84, 91, 119
Third-space losses, 227, 232, 253
Thyroid cancer 103
Thyroid Function Tests,(TSH, TRH, TBG, T4, Free T4, FTI, T3, Free T3) 24, 222, 261-75
Thyroid toxicosis, 104
Thyroiditis, 264-5, 271-2, 274, 295
Thyrotoxicosis, 108, 265
Ticarcillin, 57, 62, 84, 91, 97, 135, 170, 217, 237, 254
Ticlopidine, 57, 62, 84, 91, 97, 119, 135, 237, 255, 278
Timolol, 57, 62, 84, 91, 97, 135, 159, 170, 210, 216, 278
Tinzaparin, 57,84, 97
Tobramycin, 57, 84, 91, 97, 105, 135, 194, 198, 217, 237, 255
Tocainide, 57, 62, 84, 91
Tocopherols, 289
Tolazamide, 57, 62, 84, 91, 160
Tolazoline, 57, 62, 84, 91, 135
Tolbutamide, 57, 62, 84, 91, 120, 159, 160, 172, 237
Tolcapone, 57, 62, 84, 91, 119, 120, 128, 159
Tolmetin, 57, 62, 84, 91,92, 97, 194, 237
Topotecan, 57, 84, 91
Toremifene, 57, 62, 85, 91, 105
Torsemide, 110, 198, 219, 257
Total Iron Binding Capacity (TIBC), 42, 51, 142-3, 178, 181, 186-90, 299

Total Lymphocyte Count, 291
Total Protein, 220-37
Toxemia, 139, 234, 256, 258
Toxic shock syndrome, 81, 104
Tramadol, 57, 62, 84, 91, 135, 237
Trandolapril, 57, 84, 91, 97, 135, 216
Transferrin Saturation, 186-90
Transferrin, 24, 38-9, 142, 186-90, 228
Transfusions, 28, 145-6, 149, 187-9
Transplant rejection, 193, 202, 215, 235, 293
Tranylcypromine, 57, 84, 91
Trastuzumab, 57, 62, 84, 91, 105, 160, 198, 255
Trauma, 78, 81, 88, 92, 98, 100, 123, 125-7, 132-3, 146, 155, 169, 192, 215, 227, 235, 264, 279, 288, 292-5
Trazodone, 120
Tretinoin, 57, 62, 84, 91, 127, 135, 278
Triamcinolone, 110, 124, 159, 170, 219, 257
Triamterene, 77, 97, 110, 113, 135, 150, 159, 198, 216, 217, 257, 295
Triazolam, 57, 62, 91, 135, 159, 237
Trichlormethiazide, 57, 84, 91, 105, 110, 159, 217, 257, 278
Trifluoperazine, 57, 62, 84-5, 91, 119, 159, 237
Triglycerides, 24, 115-7, 276-278
Trimethobenzamide, 91
Trimethoprim, 57, 62, 84, 91, 97, 113, 128, 131, 135, 137, 140, 150, 159, 160, 216-7, 219, 255, 257
Trimetrexate, 57, 62, 84, 91, 97, 105, 135, 159, 255
Trimipramine, 57, 62, 84, 91, 124, 159, 160, 255
Trioxsalen, 57, 62, 84, 91
Triptorelin, 57, 84, 91
Troglitazone, 57, 62, 84, 119, 128, 160, 278
Troleandomycin, 57, 62, 84, 91, 266
Troleandomycin, 57, 62, 84, 91, 266
Tromethamine, 65, 135, 160, 216
Troponin , 279
Trovafloxacin, 57, 62, 84, 97, 135, 255
Tuberculosis, 100, 103-4, 139, 146, 231, 296
Tubocurarine, 128
Tubulointerstitial disease, 257
Ulcerative colitis, 44, 59, 149, 296, 299
Uracil mustard, , 57, 62, 84, 91
Uremia, 46, 80, 121, 141-3, 193, 205, 296
Ureteral obstruction, 95
Ureterosigmoidostomy, 64
Urinary obstruction, 95
Urinary tract infection, 53, 100
Urine Specific Gravity, 33, 252, 258
Urochromes, 92
Ursodiol, 57, 62, 84, 85, 91, 92, 120, 135, 159
Valproic acid, 57, 62, 65, 85, 91-2, 120, 135, 146, 159-60, 194, 254-5, 266, 271, 273, 275
Valsartan, 57, 85, 135, 216

Vancomycin, 97, 135, 237
Vasculitis syndrome, 100
Vasopressin, 97, 123, 128, 135, 194, 203, 255
Vegetarianism, 149
Venlafaxine, 57, 62, 85, 91, 97, 119, 135, 159, 170, 210-1, 216-7, 237, 255
Verapamil, 57, 62, 85, 91, 97, 120, 159-60, 176, 194, 203, 237, 257, 278
Vidarabine, 57, 62, 85, 91, 159, 217, 255
Vincristine, 255, 257
Vinorelbine, 255, 257
Viomycin, 219
Vitamin A, Retinol, 57, 85, 91, 119, 140, 221, 280-2
Vitamin B$_6$, 80, 149, 283-4
Vitamin B$_{12}$, 22, 43-6, 147, 215, 247-9, 285-6
Vitamin D, 59, 62, 97, 103-5, 108, 110, 119, 135, 209-10, 287-8
Vitamin E, 119, 175, 254, 289-90
Vitamin K, 91, 110, 172, 239
VLDL, 23, 114-21
Volume depletion, 32, 256
Vomiting, 31, 33, 76-8, 112, 196-7, 210, 214, 253, 258-60
Von Gierke's disease, 156, 167
Voriconazole, 91, 198
Waldenström's macroglobulinemia, 230
Warfarin, 57, 62, 85, 91, 238, 278
Water overload, 156
Weight loss surgery, 41, 47-9, 165, 298
Werner's syndrome, 70, 118, 277
Wernicke-Korsakoff syndrome, 260
Whipple's disease, 166
White Blood Cells (WBC), 29, 147, 177, 291-7
Wilson's disease, 229, 235
Wounds, 36, 214, 298
Xanthomatosis, 118
X-chromosome linked autosomal anemias, 241
Xerophthalmia, 280-1
Zafirlukast, 91
Zalcitabine, 57, 62, 85, 91, 97, 105, 128, 159, 198, 216-7, 237, 254-5, 278
Zidovudine, 57, 62, 85, 91, 128, 135, 159
Zileuton, 57, 85
Zinc, 59, 62, 91, 221, 298-9
Ziprasidone, 91, 159
Zoledronic acid, 105, 110, 135, 198, 211
Zollinger-Ellison syndrome, 239, 286
Zolmitriptan, 57, 62, 85, 91, 159
Zolpidem, 57, 62, 85, 91, 97, 119, 140, 159